Mometrix
TEST PREPARATION

CRT® & RRT®
Exam Secrets Study Guide

AF834646

Dear Future Exam Success Story

First of all, **THANK YOU** for purchasing Mometrix study materials!

Second, congratulations! You are one of the few determined test-takers who are committed to doing whatever it takes to excel on your exam. **You have come to the right place.** We developed these study materials with one goal in mind: to deliver you the information you need in a format that's concise and easy to use.

In addition to optimizing your guide for the content of the test, we've outlined our recommended steps for breaking down the preparation process into small, attainable goals so you can make sure you stay on track.

We've also analyzed the entire test-taking process, identifying the most common pitfalls and showing how you can overcome them and be ready for any curveball the test throws you.

Standardized testing is one of the biggest obstacles on your road to success, which only increases the importance of doing well in the high-pressure, high-stakes environment of test day. Your results on this test could have a significant impact on your future, and this guide provides the information and practical advice to help you achieve your full potential on test day.

Your success is our success

We would love to hear from you! If you would like to share the story of your exam success or if you have any questions or comments in regard to our products, please contact us at **800-673-8175** or **support@mometrix.com**.

Thanks again for your business and we wish you continued success!

Sincerely,
The Mometrix Test Preparation Team

Need more help? Check out our flashcards at:
http://MometrixFlashcards.com/RRT

Written and edited by the Mometrix Exam Secrets Test Prep Team
Printed in the United States of America

TABLE OF CONTENTS

Introduction

Thank you for purchasing this resource! You have made the choice to prepare yourself for a test that could have a huge impact on your future, and this guide is designed to help you be fully ready for test day. Obviously, it's important to have a solid understanding of the test material, but you also need to be prepared for the unique environment and stressors of the test, so that you can perform to the best of your abilities.

For this purpose, the first section that appears in this guide is the **Secret Keys**. We've devoted countless hours to meticulously researching what works and what doesn't, and we've boiled down our findings to the five most impactful steps you can take to improve your performance on the test. We start at the beginning with study planning and move through the preparation process, all the way to the testing strategies that will help you get the most out of what you know when you're finally sitting in front of the test.

We recommend that you start preparing for your test as far in advance as possible. However, if you've bought this guide as a last-minute study resource and only have a few days before your test, we recommend that you skip over the first two Secret Keys since they address a long-term study plan.

If you struggle with **test anxiety**, we strongly encourage you to check out our recommendations for how you can overcome it. Test anxiety is a formidable foe, but it can be beaten, and we want to make sure you have the tools you need to defeat it.

Secret Key #1 – Plan Big, Study Small

There's a lot riding on your performance. If you want to ace this test, you're going to need to keep your skills sharp and the material fresh in your mind. You need a plan that lets you review everything you need to know while still fitting in your schedule. We'll break this strategy down into three categories.

Information Organization

Start with the information you already have: the official test outline. From this, you can make a complete list of all the concepts you need to cover before the test. Organize these concepts into groups that can be studied together, and create a list of any related vocabulary you need to learn so you can brush up on any difficult terms. You'll want to keep this vocabulary list handy once you actually start studying since you may need to add to it along the way.

Time Management

Once you have your set of study concepts, decide how to spread them out over the time you have left before the test. Break your study plan into small, clear goals so you have a manageable task for each day and know exactly what you're doing. Then just focus on one small step at a time. When you manage your time this way, you don't need to spend hours at a time studying. Studying a small block of content for a short period each day helps you retain information better and avoid stressing over how much you have left to do. You can relax knowing that you have a plan to cover everything in time. In order for this strategy to be effective though, you have to start studying early and stick to your schedule. Avoid the exhaustion and futility that comes from last-minute cramming!

Study Environment

The environment you study in has a big impact on your learning. Studying in a coffee shop, while probably more enjoyable, is not likely to be as fruitful as studying in a quiet room. It's important to keep distractions to a minimum. You're only planning to study for a short block of time, so make the most of it. Don't pause to check your phone or get up to find a snack. It's also important to **avoid multitasking**. Research has consistently shown that multitasking will make your studying dramatically less effective. Your study area should also be comfortable and well-lit so you don't have the distraction of straining your eyes or sitting on an uncomfortable chair.

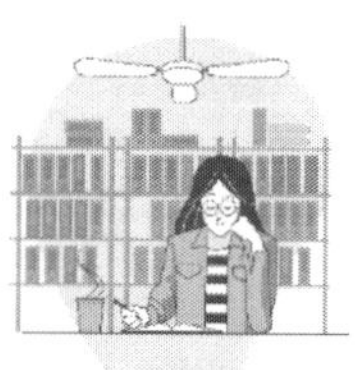

The time of day you study is also important. You want to be rested and alert. Don't wait until just before bedtime. Study when you'll be most likely to comprehend and remember. Even better, if you know what time of day your test will be, set that time aside for study. That way your brain will be used to working on that subject at that specific time and you'll have a better chance of recalling information.

Finally, it can be helpful to team up with others who are studying for the same test. Your actual studying should be done in as isolated an environment as possible, but the work of organizing the information and setting up the study plan can be divided up. In between study sessions, you can discuss with your teammates the concepts that you're all studying and quiz each other on the details. Just be sure that your teammates are as serious about the test as you are. If you find that your study time is being replaced with social time, you might need to find a new team.

Secret Key #2 – Make Your Studying Count

You're devoting a lot of time and effort to preparing for this test, so you want to be absolutely certain it will pay off. This means doing more than just reading the content and hoping you can remember it on test day. It's important to make every minute of study count. There are two main areas you can focus on to make your studying count.

Retention

It doesn't matter how much time you study if you can't remember the material. You need to make sure you are retaining the concepts. To check your retention of the information you're learning, try recalling it at later times with minimal prompting. Try carrying around flashcards and glance at one or two from time to time or ask a friend who's also studying for the test to quiz you.

To enhance your retention, look for ways to put the information into practice so that you can apply it rather than simply recalling it. If you're using the information in practical ways, it will be much easier to remember. Similarly, it helps to solidify a concept in your mind if you're not only reading it to yourself but also explaining it to someone else. Ask a friend to let you teach them about a concept you're a little shaky on (or speak aloud to an imaginary audience if necessary). As you try to summarize, define, give examples, and answer your friend's questions, you'll understand the concepts better and they will stay with you longer. Finally, step back for a big picture view and ask yourself how each piece of information fits with the whole subject. When you link the different concepts together and see them working together as a whole, it's easier to remember the individual components.

Finally, practice showing your work on any multi-step problems, even if you're just studying. Writing out each step you take to solve a problem will help solidify the process in your mind, and you'll be more likely to remember it during the test.

Modality

Modality simply refers to the means or method by which you study. Choosing a study modality that fits your own individual learning style is crucial. No two people learn best in exactly the same way, so it's important to know your strengths and use them to your advantage.

For example, if you learn best by visualization, focus on visualizing a concept in your mind and draw an image or a diagram. Try color-coding your notes, illustrating them, or creating symbols that will trigger your mind to recall a learned concept. If you learn best by hearing or discussing information, find a study partner who learns the same way or read aloud to yourself. Think about how to put the information in your own words. Imagine that you are giving a lecture on the topic and record yourself so you can listen to it later.

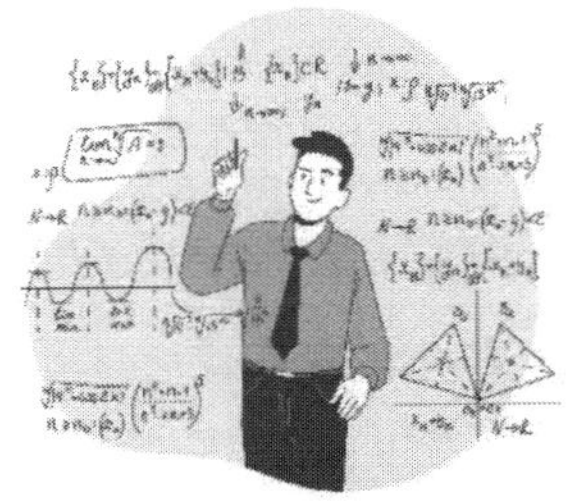

For any learning style, flashcards can be helpful. Organize the information so you can take advantage of spare moments to review. Underline key words or phrases. Use different colors for different categories. Mnemonic devices (such as creating a short list in which every item starts with the same letter) can also help with retention. Find what works best for you and use it to store the information in your mind most effectively and easily.

Secret Key #3 – Practice the Right Way

Your success on test day depends not only on how many hours you put into preparing, but also on whether you prepared the right way. It's good to check along the way to see if your studying is paying off. One of the most effective ways to do this is by taking practice tests to evaluate your progress. Practice tests are useful because they show exactly where you need to improve. Every time you take a practice test, pay special attention to these three groups of questions:

- The questions you got wrong
- The questions you had to guess on, even if you guessed right
- The questions you found difficult or slow to work through

This will show you exactly what your weak areas are, and where you need to devote more study time. Ask yourself why each of these questions gave you trouble. Was it because you didn't understand the material? Was it because you didn't remember the vocabulary? Do you need more repetitions on this type of question to build speed and confidence? Dig into those questions and figure out how you can strengthen your weak areas as you go back to review the material.

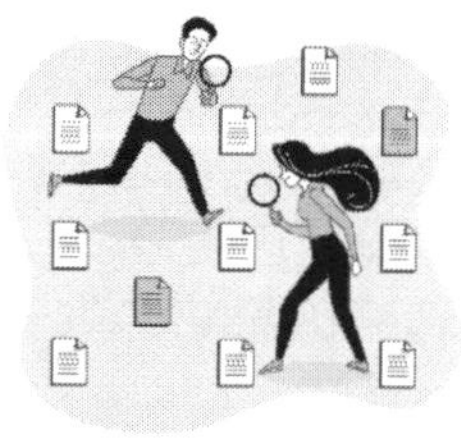

Additionally, many practice tests have a section explaining the answer choices. It can be tempting to read the explanation and think that you now have a good understanding of the concept. However, an explanation likely only covers part of the question's broader context. Even if the explanation makes perfect sense, **go back and investigate** every concept related to the question until you're positive you have a thorough understanding.

As you go along, keep in mind that the practice test is just that: practice. Memorizing these questions and answers will not be very helpful on the actual test because it is unlikely to have any of the same exact questions. If you only know the right answers to the sample questions, you won't be prepared for the real thing. **Study the concepts** until you understand them fully, and then you'll be able to answer any question that shows up on the test.

It's important to wait on the practice tests until you're ready. If you take a test on your first day of study, you may be overwhelmed by the amount of material covered and how much you need to learn. Work up to it gradually.

On test day, you'll need to be prepared for answering questions, managing your time, and using the test-taking strategies you've learned. It's a lot to balance, like a mental marathon that will have a big impact on your future. Like training for a marathon, you'll need to start slowly and work your way up. When test day arrives, you'll be ready.

Start with the strategies you've read in the first two Secret Keys—plan your course and study in the way that works best for you. If you have time, consider using multiple study resources to get different approaches to the same concepts. It can be helpful to see difficult concepts from more than one angle. Then find a good source for practice tests. Many times, the test website will suggest potential study resources or provide sample tests.

Practice Test Strategy

If you're able to find at least three practice tests, we recommend this strategy:

Untimed and Open-Book Practice

Take the first test with no time constraints and with your notes and study guide handy. Take your time and focus on applying the strategies you've learned.

Timed and Open-Book Practice

Take the second practice test open-book as well, but set a timer and practice pacing yourself to finish in time.

Timed and Closed-Book Practice

Take any other practice tests as if it were test day. Set a timer and put away your study materials. Sit at a table or desk in a quiet room, imagine yourself at the testing center, and answer questions as quickly and accurately as possible.

Keep repeating timed and closed-book tests on a regular basis until you run out of practice tests or it's time for the actual test. Your mind will be ready for the schedule and stress of test day, and you'll be able to focus on recalling the material you've learned.

Secret Key #4 – Pace Yourself

Once you're fully prepared for the material on the test, your biggest challenge on test day will be managing your time. Just knowing that the clock is ticking can make you panic even if you have plenty of time left. Work on pacing yourself so you can build confidence against the time constraints of the exam. Pacing is a difficult skill to master, especially in a high-pressure environment, so **practice is vital**.

Set time expectations for your pace based on how much time is available. For example, if a section has 60 questions and the time limit is 30 minutes, you know you have to average 30 seconds or less per question in order to answer them all. Although 30 seconds is the hard limit, set 25 seconds per question as your goal, so you reserve extra time to spend on harder questions. When you budget extra time for the harder questions, you no longer have any reason to stress when those questions take longer to answer.

Don't let this time expectation distract you from working through the test at a calm, steady pace, but keep it in mind so you don't spend too much time on any one question. Recognize that taking extra time on one question you don't understand may keep you from answering two that you do understand later in the test. If your time limit for a question is up and you're still not sure of the answer, mark it and move on, and come back to it later if the time and the test format allow. If the testing format doesn't allow you to return to earlier questions, just make an educated guess; then put it out of your mind and move on.

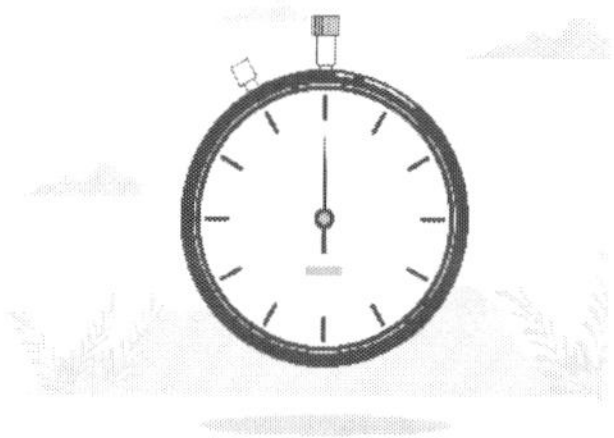

On the easier questions, be careful not to rush. It may seem wise to hurry through them so you have more time for the challenging ones, but it's not worth missing one if you know the concept and just didn't take the time to read the question fully. Work efficiently but make sure you understand the question and have looked at all of the answer choices, since more than one may seem right at first.

Even if you're paying attention to the time, you may find yourself a little behind at some point. You should speed up to get back on track, but do so wisely. Don't panic; just take a few seconds less on each question until you're caught up. Don't guess without thinking, but do look through the answer choices and eliminate any you know are wrong. If you can get down to two choices, it is often worthwhile to guess from those. Once you've chosen an answer, move on and don't dwell on any that you skipped or had to hurry through. If a question was taking too long, chances are it was one of the harder ones, so you weren't as likely to get it right anyway.

On the other hand, if you find yourself getting ahead of schedule, it may be beneficial to slow down a little. The more quickly you work, the more likely you are to make a careless mistake that will affect your score. You've budgeted time for each question, so don't be afraid to spend that time. Practice an efficient but careful pace to get the most out of the time you have.

Secret Key #5 – Have a Plan for Guessing

When you're taking the test, you may find yourself stuck on a question. Some of the answer choices seem better than others, but you don't see the one answer choice that is obviously correct. What do you do?

The scenario described above is very common, yet most test takers have not effectively prepared for it. Developing and practicing a plan for guessing may be one of the single most effective uses of your time as you get ready for the exam.

In developing your plan for guessing, there are three questions to address:

- When should you start the guessing process?
- How should you narrow down the choices?
- Which answer should you choose?

When to Start the Guessing Process

Unless your plan for guessing is to select C every time (which, despite its merits, is not what we recommend), you need to leave yourself enough time to apply your answer elimination strategies. Since you have a limited amount of time for each question, that means that if you're going to give yourself the best shot at guessing correctly, you have to decide quickly whether or not you will guess.

Of course, the best-case scenario is that you don't have to guess at all, so first, see if you can answer the question based on your knowledge of the subject and basic reasoning skills. Focus on the key words in the question and try to jog your memory of related topics. Give yourself a chance to bring the knowledge to mind, but once you realize that you don't have (or you can't access) the knowledge you need to answer the question, it's time to start the guessing process.

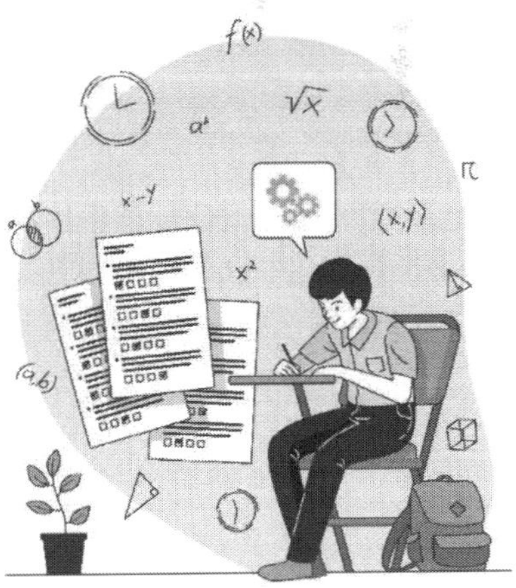

It's almost always better to start the guessing process too early than too late. It only takes a few seconds to remember something and answer the question from knowledge. Carefully eliminating wrong answer choices takes longer. Plus, going through the process of eliminating answer choices can actually help jog your memory.

Summary: Start the guessing process as soon as you decide that you can't answer the question based on your knowledge.

How to Narrow Down the Choices

The next chapter in this book (**Test-Taking Strategies**) includes a wide range of strategies for how to approach questions and how to look for answer choices to eliminate. You will definitely want to read those carefully, practice them, and figure out which ones work best for you. Here though, we're going to address a mindset rather than a particular strategy.

Your odds of guessing an answer correctly depend on how many options you are choosing from.

Number of options left	5	4	3	2	1
Odds of guessing correctly	20%	25%	33%	50%	100%

You can see from this chart just how valuable it is to be able to eliminate incorrect answers and make an educated guess, but there are two things that many test takers do that cause them to miss out on the benefits of guessing:

- Accidentally eliminating the correct answer
- Selecting an answer based on an impression

We'll look at the first one here, and the second one in the next section.

To avoid accidentally eliminating the correct answer, we recommend a thought exercise called **the $5 challenge**. In this challenge, you only eliminate an answer choice from contention if you are willing to bet $5 on it being wrong. Why $5? Five dollars is a small but not insignificant amount of money. It's an amount you could afford to lose but wouldn't want to throw away. And while losing $5 once might not hurt too much, doing it twenty times will set you back $100. In the same way, each small decision you make—eliminating a choice here, guessing on a question there—won't by itself impact your score very much, but when you put them all together, they can make a big difference. By holding each answer choice elimination decision to a higher standard, you can reduce the risk of accidentally eliminating the correct answer.

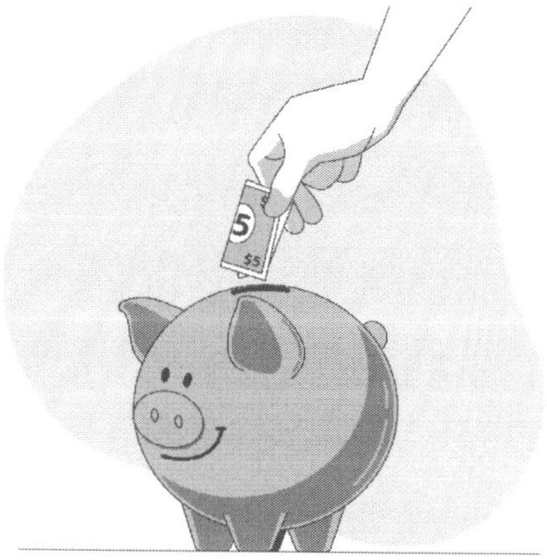

The $5 challenge can also be applied in a positive sense: If you are willing to bet $5 that an answer choice *is* correct, go ahead and mark it as correct.

Summary: Only eliminate an answer choice if you are willing to bet $5 that it is wrong.

Which Answer to Choose

You're taking the test. You've run into a hard question and decided you'll have to guess. You've eliminated all the answer choices you're willing to bet $5 on. Now you have to pick an answer. Why do we even need to talk about this? Why can't you just pick whichever one you feel like when the time comes?

The answer to these questions is that if you don't come into the test with a plan, you'll rely on your impression to select an answer choice, and if you do that, you risk falling into a trap. The test writers know that everyone who takes their test will be guessing on some of the questions, so they intentionally write wrong answer choices to seem plausible. You still have to pick an answer though, and if the wrong answer choices are designed to look right, how can you ever be sure that you're not falling for their trap? The best solution we've found to this dilemma is to take the decision out of your hands entirely. Here is the process we recommend:

Once you've eliminated any choices that you are confident (willing to bet $5) are wrong, select the first remaining choice as your answer.

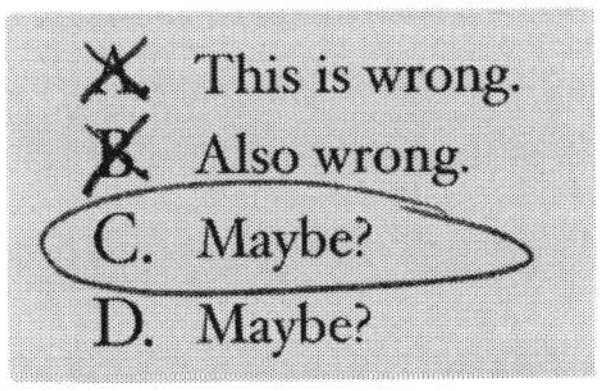

Whether you choose to select the first remaining choice, the second, or the last, the important thing is that you use some preselected standard. Using this approach guarantees that you will not be enticed into selecting an answer choice that looks right, because you are not basing your decision on how the answer choices look.

This is not meant to make you question your knowledge. Instead, it is to help you recognize the difference between your knowledge and your impressions. There's a huge difference between thinking an answer is right because of what you know, and thinking an answer is right because it looks or sounds like it should be right.

Summary: To ensure that your selection is appropriately random, make a predetermined selection from among all answer choices you have not eliminated.

Test-Taking Strategies

This section contains a list of test-taking strategies that you may find helpful as you work through the test. By taking what you know and applying logical thought, you can maximize your chances of answering any question correctly!

It is very important to realize that every question is different and every person is different: no single strategy will work on every question, and no single strategy will work for every person. That's why we've included all of them here, so you can try them out and determine which ones work best for different types of questions and which ones work best for you.

Question Strategies

☑ Read Carefully

Read the question and the answer choices carefully. Don't miss the question because you misread the terms. You have plenty of time to read each question thoroughly and make sure you understand what is being asked. Yet a happy medium must be attained, so don't waste too much time. You must read carefully and efficiently.

☑ Contextual Clues

Look for contextual clues. If the question includes a word you are not familiar with, look at the immediate context for some indication of what the word might mean. Contextual clues can often give you all the information you need to decipher the meaning of an unfamiliar word. Even if you can't determine the meaning, you may be able to narrow down the possibilities enough to make a solid guess at the answer to the question.

☑ Prefixes

If you're having trouble with a word in the question or answer choices, try dissecting it. Take advantage of every clue that the word might include. Prefixes can be a huge help. Usually, they allow you to determine a basic meaning. *Pre-* means before, *post-* means after, *pro-* is positive, *de-* is negative. From prefixes, you can get an idea of the general meaning of the word and try to put it into context.

☑ Hedge Words

Watch out for critical hedge words, such as *likely, may, can, often, almost, mostly, usually, generally, rarely,* and *sometimes.* Question writers insert these hedge phrases to cover every possibility. Often an answer choice will be wrong simply because it leaves no room for exception. Be on guard for answer choices that have definitive words such as *exactly* and *always.*

☑ Switchback Words

Stay alert for *switchbacks.* These are the words and phrases frequently used to alert you to shifts in thought. The most common switchback words are *but, although,* and *however.* Others include *nevertheless, on the other hand, even though, while, in spite of, despite,* and *regardless of.* Switchback words are important to catch because they can change the direction of the question or an answer choice.

☑ Face Value

When in doubt, use common sense. Accept the situation in the problem at face value. Don't read too much into it. These problems will not require you to make wild assumptions. If you have to go beyond creativity and warp time or space in order to have an answer choice fit the question, then you should move on and consider the other answer choices. These are normal problems rooted in reality. The applicable relationship or explanation may not be readily apparent, but it is there for you to figure out. Use your common sense to interpret anything that isn't clear.

Answer Choice Strategies

☑ Answer Selection

The most thorough way to pick an answer choice is to identify and eliminate wrong answers until only one is left, then confirm it is the correct answer. Sometimes an answer choice may immediately seem right, but be careful. The test writers will usually put more than one reasonable answer choice on each question, so take a second to read all of them and make sure that the other choices are not equally obvious. As long as you have time left, it is better to read every answer choice than to pick the first one that looks right without checking the others.

☑ Answer Choice Families

An answer choice family consists of two (in rare cases, three) answer choices that are very similar in construction and cannot all be true at the same time. If you see two answer choices that are direct opposites or parallels, one of them is usually the correct answer. For instance, if one answer choice says that quantity x increases and another either says that quantity x decreases (opposite) or says that quantity y increases (parallel), then those answer choices would fall into the same family. An answer choice that doesn't match the construction of the answer choice family is more likely to be incorrect. Most questions will not have answer choice families, but when they do appear, you should be prepared to recognize them.

☑ Eliminate Answers

Eliminate answer choices as soon as you realize they are wrong, but make sure you consider all possibilities. If you are eliminating answer choices and realize that the last one you are left with is also wrong, don't panic. Start over and consider each choice again. There may be something you missed the first time that you will realize on the second pass.

☑ Avoid Fact Traps

Don't be distracted by an answer choice that is factually true but doesn't answer the question. You are looking for the choice that answers the question. Stay focused on what the question is asking for so you don't accidentally pick an answer that is true but incorrect. Always go back to the question and make sure the answer choice you've selected actually answers the question and is not merely a true statement.

☑ Extreme Statements

In general, you should avoid answers that put forth extreme actions as standard practice or proclaim controversial ideas as established fact. An answer choice that states the "process should be used in certain situations, if..." is much more likely to be correct than one that states the "process should be discontinued completely." The first is a calm rational statement and doesn't even make a definitive, uncompromising stance, using a hedge word *if* to provide wiggle room, whereas the second choice is far more extreme.

⊘ Benchmark

As you read through the answer choices and you come across one that seems to answer the question well, mentally select that answer choice. This is not your final answer, but it's the one that will help you evaluate the other answer choices. The one that you selected is your benchmark or standard for judging each of the other answer choices. Every other answer choice must be compared to your benchmark. That choice is correct until proven otherwise by another answer choice beating it. If you find a better answer, then that one becomes your new benchmark. Once you've decided that no other choice answers the question as well as your benchmark, you have your final answer.

⊘ Predict the Answer

Before you even start looking at the answer choices, it is often best to try to predict the answer. When you come up with the answer on your own, it is easier to avoid distractions and traps because you will know exactly what to look for. The right answer choice is unlikely to be word-for-word what you came up with, but it should be a close match. Even if you are confident that you have the right answer, you should still take the time to read each option before moving on.

General Strategies

⊘ Tough Questions

If you are stumped on a problem or it appears too hard or too difficult, don't waste time. Move on! Remember though, if you can quickly check for obviously incorrect answer choices, your chances of guessing correctly are greatly improved. Before you completely give up, at least try to knock out a couple of possible answers. Eliminate what you can and then guess at the remaining answer choices before moving on.

⊘ Check Your Work

Since you will probably not know every term listed and the answer to every question, it is important that you get credit for the ones that you do know. Don't miss any questions through careless mistakes. If at all possible, try to take a second to look back over your answer selection and make sure you've selected the correct answer choice and haven't made a costly careless mistake (such as marking an answer choice that you didn't mean to mark). This quick double check should more than pay for itself in caught mistakes for the time it costs.

⊘ Pace Yourself

It's easy to be overwhelmed when you're looking at a page full of questions; your mind is confused and full of random thoughts, and the clock is ticking down faster than you would like. Calm down and maintain the pace that you have set for yourself. Especially as you get down to the last few minutes of the test, don't let the small numbers on the clock make you panic. As long as you are on track by monitoring your pace, you are guaranteed to have time for each question.

⊘ Don't Rush

It is very easy to make errors when you are in a hurry. Maintaining a fast pace in answering questions is pointless if it makes you miss questions that you would have gotten right otherwise. Test writers like to include distracting information and wrong answers that seem right. Taking a little extra time to avoid careless mistakes can make all the difference in your test score. Find a pace that allows you to be confident in the answers that you select.

✓ Keep Moving

Panicking will not help you pass the test, so do your best to stay calm and keep moving. Taking deep breaths and going through the answer elimination steps you practiced can help to break through a stress barrier and keep your pace.

Final Notes

The combination of a solid foundation of content knowledge and the confidence that comes from practicing your plan for applying that knowledge is the key to maximizing your performance on test day. As your foundation of content knowledge is built up and strengthened, you'll find that the strategies included in this chapter become more and more effective in helping you quickly sift through the distractions and traps of the test to isolate the correct answer.

Now that you're preparing to move forward into the test content chapters of this book, be sure to keep your goal in mind. As you read, think about how you will be able to apply this information on the test. If you've already seen sample questions for the test and you have an idea of the question format and style, try to come up with questions of your own that you can answer based on what you're reading. This will give you valuable practice applying your knowledge in the same ways you can expect to on test day.

Good luck and good studying!

Patient Data

Evaluate Data in the Patient Record

Complete Blood Count (CBC)

A complete blood count is comprised of the number of red blood cells, white blood cells, and platelets. It is a blood draw that is done as part of an initial workup for many health issues, including suspected infection and bleeding. The normal range for these components can be slightly different for men and women. For women, a normal red blood cell count ranges from $3.8–5.2 \times 10^6$ mcl, hemoglobin ranges from 11.7–15.7 g/dl, and hematocrit ranges from 35–47%. For men, red blood cell count ranges from $4.4–5.9 \times 10^6$ mcl, hemoglobin ranges from 13.3–17.7 g/dl, and hematocrit ranges from 40–52%. White blood cell count for both men and women ranges from $3.9–11.7 \times 10^3$ mcl. Numbers outside of the normal ranges can indicate infection, acute blood loss, or bone marrow disease. Results should be correlated with the patient's presenting symptoms and assessment.

Apgar Score

The Apgar score is an assessment tool that is used to monitor how a newborn is transitioning from intrauterine to extrauterine life. An infant is assigned a score from 0 to 10, with normal being 7 or higher. The newborn is scored at 1, 5, and 10 minutes after birth. If after 10 minutes the infant is still not transitioning effectively, an Apgar will continue to be assigned every 5 minutes as needed until a score of 7 is reached. Apgar scoring has five assessment areas and includes the newborn's appearance, pulse, grimace, activity and reflex, and respirations, with a score of 0-2 assigned for each of the 5 areas. The scores for each area are added together and the sum represents the infant's overall Apgar score.

Surfactant

Surfactant is a substance secreted into the alveoli by Type II pneumocytes. Surfactant is composed of phospholipids and proteins. The purpose of surfactant is to line the alveoli at the air/liquid interface and to help prevent lung collapse with each exhalation. The repelling forces in the surfactant only allow lung recoil to a certain amount, and then repel each other to keep the alveoli expanded until the next breath. When either the production or activity of surfactant is inhibited, the patient will present with respiratory distress and increasing difficulty breathing. Surfactant production is altered in infants born prior to 36 weeks gestation, as well as infants presenting with meconium aspiration syndrome. In these cases, artificial surfactant can be instilled into the lungs to support the infant until he is able to produce his own surfactant.

Arterial Blood Gas (ABG)

Arterial blood gas results involve interpreting the pH, PCO_2, PO_2, and Bicarbonate. Normal ranges for each are as follows: pH: 7.35–7.45, PCO_2: 35–45, PO_2: 80–100, HCO_3: 22–28. Interpretation of the results can be done with four steps. First, assess the pH for acidosis (<7.35) or alkalosis (>7.45). Second, assess for respiratory involvement by categorizing the CO_2. If the CO_2 is abnormal in the opposite direction of the pH abnormality, and the HCO_3 is normal, there is a primary respiratory cause. Third, assess for metabolic involvement. If HCO_3 is abnormal in the same direction of the pH abnormality, and the CO_2 is in the normal range, there is a primary metabolic cause. Finally, evaluate for any compensation. Once the primary cause of the disturbance is identified, the body will attempt to compensate by altering the other component. If the other component is also outside of the normal range, and the pH is brought back to normal, the ABG is considered compensated.

Lactate Levels

Lactate levels are drawn when there is a concern for sepsis caused by an overwhelming infection in the body. They can also be drawn in patients with inadequate perfusion to check the level of oxygenation to the tissues. The levels are most commonly added to an arterial blood gas analysis. Lactate levels are a measurement of the lactic acid in the blood. Normal lactate levels are less than 2 mmol/L. The significance of an elevated lactate level comes from the fact that lactic acid is a byproduct of anaerobic respiration. As oxygen delivery to the tissues decreases, the body must begin to use anaerobic respiration, rather than the preferred aerobic respiration. The longer the tissues are oxygen deprived, the higher the lactate level will be in the circulating blood.

Electrolyte Balance

Proper electrolyte balance is crucial for maintaining homeostasis of all body systems. A basic metabolic panel (BMP) will assess sodium, potassium, and calcium. In the cardiopulmonary system, abnormal sodium levels can be indicative of dehydration and may lead to thickened mucus in hypernatremia or congestive heart failure in hyponatremia. Abnormal potassium levels can be associated with renal disease and alcoholism in hyperkalemia or high doses of beta-agonist medication in hypokalemia. Abnormal calcium levels are consistent with diuretic therapy and lead to hypercalcemia, or pancreatitis and administration of blood products can lead to hypocalcemia. In addition, magnesium and phosphorus can be assessed with a complex metabolic panel (CMP). Magnesium abnormalities can be associated with chronic renal failure, causing hypermagnesia, or with dialysis and digestive issues in hypomagnesia. Finally, phosphorus abnormalities can be indicative of renal or liver failure in hyperphosphatemia or chronic hyperventilation syndrome in hypophosphatemia.

Cellular Fluid Composition

Normal cellular fluid is composed of a 0.9% sodium chloride solution. When a cell is placed in a fluid with the same concentration of sodium chloride, the fluid is considered to be isotonic, or the same tonicity. If a cell is placed in a fluid with higher tonicity, or higher sodium concentration, the fluid is considered to be hypertonic. If a cell is placed in a fluid with lower tonicity, or lower sodium concentration, the fluid is considered to be hypotonic. Since water moves through the cell wall in order to balance the tonicity inside and outside the cell, a hypertonic solution will draw water out of the cell, causing the cell to shrink. When placed in a hypotonic solution, water will move into the cell, causing it to enlarge and eventually burst (lyse).

Respiratory Failure

Type I respiratory failure, or hypoxemic respiratory failure, is considered failure to oxygenate. Primary causes for this type of respiratory failure include hypoventilation of gas exchange units, disruption in the normal ventilation/ perfusion ratios, inability of gas to diffuse into the capillaries, or shunting of blood past the gas exchange units of the lungs. In addition, inhaling a lower oxygen concentration or a low mixed venous saturation can lower arterial oxygen content. Type II respiratory failure, or hypercapnic respiratory failure, is a failure to ventilate. Primary causes of type II respiratory failure include decreased ventilation caused by chronic respiratory disorders such as asthma, COPD, or emphysema, increased carbon dioxide production in the body, neurological disorders affecting the respiratory control center of the brain or spinal cord, and muscular disorders affecting respiratory muscle strength.

Advance Directives and DNR Orders

There are two types of advance directives commonly used: a durable power of attorney and a living will. A durable power of attorney is an official document that states who has the power to make medical decisions for a patient if he becomes incapacitated or unable to make medical decisions for himself. In contrast, a living will states specifically what a person wants done in the event he becomes incapacitated or unable to state what he wants in terms of procedures or life-prolonging interventions. In addition, a do not resuscitate order states what the person would like done in the event that he goes into cardiac arrest. For example, a do not resuscitate order may state that a person can become intubated, but no chest compressions. The wishes within a do not resuscitate order can be a part of a person's living will.

Impact That Prematurity and Postmaturity Can Have on a Newborn's Lung Function

Premature and postmature infants can be at a greater risk for short- and long-term deficiencies in lung function. Premature infants are at risk for respiratory distress syndrome from lack of surfactant at birth, friable lung tissue from underdevelopment, and lung scarring from long-term mechanical ventilation and high levels of inspired oxygen due to the underdevelopment of the lungs and pulmonary vasculature. Conversely, postterm neonates are at high risk of meconium aspiration syndrome, causing inactivation of surfactant and inflammation of the lung tissue. In addition, meconium may block some small airways and not others, leading to overdistention and pneumothorax in one area while other lung units collapse. The disruption in normal rising oxygen levels at birth can also affect transitioning to extrauterine circulation that can lead to Persistent Pulmonary Hypertension of the Newborn (PPHN).

Effect of Anemia on Oxygen Content

Anemia refers to a decrease in the number of circulating red blood cells. Red blood cells contain the iron-rich hemoglobin that binds to and carries oxygen. Since anemia lowers the blood's capacity to carry oxygen in the blood, there is less oxygen carried to the tissues, and therefore less oxygen available for necessary metabolic processes. When an anemic patient has a pulse ox placed, the SpO_2 may still read normal (>92%) since it is measuring a percentage of the hemoglobin being carried in the blood, not considering the decrease in hemoglobin available. Therefore, a patient with half of the normal red blood cells may read a saturation of 100%, but the body is only receiving half of the oxygen it would with a normal red blood cell count.

Impact of Anion Gap on Blood Gas Interpretation

Anion gap is a calculation of the balance of cations and anions in the blood. Anion gap is equal to the sodium level minus the chloride level, plus the bicarbonate level. A normal anion gap is between 9 and 14 mEq/L. If the anion gap is greater than 14, metabolic acidosis occurs (pH <7.35). An increase in anion gap can be caused by too much acid being produced in the body, ingestion of an acid, or loss of bicarbonate through the gastrointestinal system. The respiratory system will attempt to compensate for this increased anion gap through hyperventilation to return the pH level back to a normal range. An increase in bicarbonate can lead to a drop in anion gap below 9 and is most commonly caused by vomiting, use of diuretics, or an over infusion of sodium bicarbonate. The increased bicarbonate leads to metabolic alkalosis (pH >7.45).

Inspection of Chest Tube Drainage Systems

Chest tubes are designed to drain fluid and/or air from the pleural space in the chest cavity. When assessing a chest tube drainage system, or a Pleur-evac system, it should be checked for functionality and ongoing drainage. The chamber that regulates pressure should be checked and adjusted to the prescribed pressure (usually -20). The Pleur-evac is connected to wall suction, but the actual suction applied to the system is adjusted via the Pleur-evac itself. Respiratory variation is a natural occurrence that should take place with each breath in the collection compartment as pleural pressures increase and decrease. If a pneumothorax is still present, bubbling in this compartment indicates an air leak. A collection compartment is also present for pleural fluid from the pleural cavity. When assessing a Pleur-evac system, it is important to check the entire system for connection integrity, including the chest tube insertion site, chest tube to Pleur-evac connection, and Pleur-evac to suction connection. The water level of the air bubbling chamber should also be checked and water replaced as needed.

Review Video: Chest Tubes
Visit mometrix.com/academy and enter code: 696975

Causes of Increased and Decreased Respiratory Compliance

Pulmonary compliance relates to the lungs' ability to stretch and relax. Pulmonary compliance can be assessed on an intubated patient by performing an end-inspiratory hold. Decreases in respiratory compliance indicate decreased ability of the patients' lungs to expand and contract. Decreased compliance can be caused from within the lungs, such as atelectasis, ARDS, pneumonia, pulmonary edema, pneumothorax or hemothorax, or diseases of the lung tissue itself, such as fibrosis. Thoracic compliance can be decreased by an increase in pressure from the abdomen, such as obesity or ascites, or deformities in the chest wall, such as a small rib cage. Increases in pulmonary compliance can be caused by reversing the diseases mentioned above, and can also be caused by pulmonary emphysema. Increases in thoracic compliance can be caused by flail chest or the removal of ribs, or by changing a patient's position to allow for greater lung expansion.

Causes of Increased and Decreased Respiratory Resistance

Pulmonary resistance is the resistance to airflow through the airways and is mostly based on the size and caliber of the airways. Pulmonary resistance can be influenced by multiple factors, including the chest wall, airway, and total respiratory resistance. Airway resistance can be calculated using airway opening pressure minus alveolar pressure. Increases in respiratory resistance can be caused by secretions that block an endotracheal tube or by the patient biting the airway. An endotracheal tube that is too small can also cause increased resistance. In addition, airway edema, bronchoconstriction, an increase in secretions, or too much gas flow can all increase resistance. Decreased airway resistance can be caused by inhaled or intravenous bronchodilators, removal of secretions, and decreasing gas flow. Increased airway resistance is often seen in patients suffering from asthma attacks or anaphylaxis.

Importance of Fluid Balance in the Critically Ill Patient

Proper fluid balance is important for a variety of reasons, including maintaining appropriate hemodynamics, electrolyte balance, and respiratory mucosa and secretion consistency and removal. Decreased fluid can create dry, thin secretions that are difficult for the patient to cough up, leading to mucus plugging and possible pneumonia. Additionally, dehydration decreases the effectiveness of the mucociliary elevator and mucus clearance. Decreased fluid balance can also reduce preload to the heart and cause hypotension. This decrease in blood pressure can impair the ventilation/perfusion ratio in the lungs and decrease oxygenation to the tissues and organs. Increased fluid balance can create too much fluid in the airways and pulmonary edema due to increased afterload. Proper fluid balance can also keep electrolytes within normal limits. When fluid is decreased, this can create a higher concentration of electrolytes, causing fluid shifts in and out of cells.

Vascular Lines

Vascular lines are important monitoring tools for patients with respiratory disorders. Arterial lines, the most common vascular lines used in respiratory therapy, are commonly placed by physicians. The vascular line provides continuous monitoring of the patient's arterial pressures, which in turn can help monitor and/or diagnose heart disorders such as right heart failure, cor pulmonale, left heart failure, valve disorders, pulmonary edema, and pulmonary hypertension. Respiratory therapists are responsible for monitoring arterial lines, observing and recording the information provided by the vascular line, and taking appropriate action to treat any unexpected adverse event or respiratory disorder. The respiratory therapist must also ensure that the line is undisturbed and patent, taking care not to displace the line during treatment.

Apnea-Hypopnea Index (AHI)

The apnea-hypopnea index is the number of apneic periods measured during a sleep study. The term apnea refers to a period of time with an absence of respiration. Apnea is commonly diagnosed after 10 seconds with the absence of respiration. In other words, if the patient does not take a breath within 10 seconds, a period of apnea has taken place. The term hypopnea refers to an insufficient respiration as a result of taking shallow tidal volumes or having an abnormally low respiratory rate. The apnea-hypopnea index can be measured via inpatient our outpatient sleep studies. This value reflects the severity of sleep apnea based on the number of apneic episodes and insufficient ventilation taking place during the exam. A normal apnea-hypopnea index value is less than 5. An apnea-hypopnea index of 5–15 is indicative of mild sleep apnea, whereas an index of 16–30 is considered to be moderate sleep apnea. If the apnea-hypopnea index is greater than 30, the patient has severe sleep apnea.

Perform Clinical Assessment

Expected X-Ray Findings for Airspace Disease and Interstitial Disease

The ability to differentiate between disease processes via x-ray is a first step in getting the patient on the right path for diagnosis and appropriate treatment. An x-ray is usually the first diagnostic imaging performed when there is suspected alteration in the pulmonary system. Airspace disease can be determined by the presence of air bronchograms, "fluffy" infiltrates, and segmental or lobar differentiation. Airspace disease tends to be difficult to define to one area of the lung as it can lack clear borders. Causes of airspace disease can be acute (pneumonia, pulmonary edema, near drowning) or chronic (sarcoidosis, lymphoma). Interstitial diseases are more commonly present with nodules, cysts, and lines differentiating lobes. Causes of interstitial lung disease on x-ray include pulmonary fibrosis, sarcoidosis of the lungs, tuberculosis, and carcinoma.

Normal Physiological Airway Clearance

Normal airway clearance is caused by various aspects of the respiratory system. A thin layer of mucus lines the airways as a protective mechanism against debris and helps trap foreign objects before they enter the lower airways. Proper hydration keeps the mucosa adequately moist so it can trap foreign debris. As this debris lands in the mucus, the cilia in the respiratory tract act as an "elevator" to push the debris up to the larynx, where it can either be coughed up or swallowed and digested. An intact cough reflex is necessary for the debris to stimulate the cough, and normal muscle strength and nerve innervation of the diaphragm is required to produce a sufficiently forceful cough.

Types of Questions for a Patient Interview

In order to obtain the most thorough medical history and accurately diagnosis a patient, the healthcare professional needs to ask specific questions that pertain to the patient's history and the current illness. There are five types of pertinent questions: 1) Open-ended questions should be used to coach patients to answer in more detail, rather than a yes or no answer. 2) Closed-ended questions are used to determine precise data about the illness, such as timeline or specific symptoms. 3) Direct questions can be open or closed, but are used to gain an exact answer. 4) Indirect questions can be used to reiterate or clarify something a patient has said or information present in the patient's chart. 5) Neutral questions can be used to move the conversation forward.

Ventilation/Perfusion Ratio

In order to maintain homeostasis, the respiratory and cardiac systems need to maintain a careful balance. The ventilation/perfusion ratio indicates that ventilation of the lungs and perfusion to the lungs are within a normal balance. A normal ventilation/perfusion ratio is equal to 0.8. A ventilation/perfusion ratio higher than normal is indicative of ventilation being too high, perfusion that is too low, or some combination of the two. This can occur because of hyperventilation (either physiological or caused by healthcare practitioners due to incorrect ventilator settings), pulmonary embolism, or hypotension. Essentially, a high ventilation/perfusion ratio means that there is more ventilation than perfusion. If the ventilation/perfusion ratio is lower than normal, then ventilation is too low, perfusion is too high, or there is some combination of the two. This can be caused by atelectasis, pneumonia, or lung disease. Whatever the cause, a low ventilation/perfusion ratio indicates that there is more perfusion than ventilation.

Normal and Abnormal Breath Sound Terms

Normal breath sounds can be divided into three types. Vesicular breath sounds are low, soft sounds that can normally be heard over the peripheral lung space. Bronchovesicular breath sounds are moderate pitch breath sounds that are normally heard in the upper lung fields. Tracheal breath sounds are higher in pitch and heard over the trachea. Abnormal breath sounds are also known as adventitious lung sounds. Wheezes are high-pitched, expiratory sounds caused by air flowing through an obstructed airway. Stridor is also high-pitched, but is usually heard on inspiration in the upper airways. Coarse crackles are caused by an excessive amount of secretions in the airway and can be heard on inspiration and expiration. Fine crackles occur late in the expiratory phase and usually occur when the peripheral airways are being "popped" back open.

Review Video: Different Types of Lung Sounds
Visit mometrix.com/academy and enter code: 765616

Identifying Cardiopulmonary Disease Through Examination of Extremities and Heart Sounds

Patients with cardiac disease can present with pulmonary symptoms, and it may be difficult to distinguish between them initially when patients have a history of both. Shortness of breath, low oxygen saturation, and tachycardia can be signs of both cardiac and pulmonary disease. Further patient examination will be necessary to pinpoint the source of the distress. Inspection of extremities can reveal edema and an increase in capillary refill time that together indicate a cardiac problem, such as congestive heart failure. In addition, heart sounds can present as muffled or distant sounds, murmurs, and arrhythmias that can assist in differentiating between the symptoms. If extremities appear normal, with little to no edema or swelling, and heart sounds appear normal or at the patient's baseline, then the origin of distress is most likely pulmonary. It is important to look at all aspects of the exam, as it is possible to have both pulmonary and cardiac disease flares at the same time.

Structures of the Heart and the Flow of Blood

Venous blood returns from the head and chest to the heart through the superior vena cava. Venous blood from the lower body returns to the heart through the inferior vena cava. The superior and inferior vessels combine to form the vena cava, which connects to the right atrium where blood flow enters. Once in the right atrium, blood is then pumped through the tricuspid valve into the right ventricle. The right ventricle pumps blood through the pulmonary valve and into the pulmonary artery. The main pulmonary artery bifurcates into the left main pulmonary artery and right main pulmonary artery, and then circulates the blood through the pulmonary vasculature for gas exchange. Oxygenated blood then returns to the left atrium through the pulmonary vein. Once in the left atrium, the blood is forced through the bicuspid valve, into the left ventricle, through the aortic valve, and out the aorta to deliver oxygenated blood to the body.

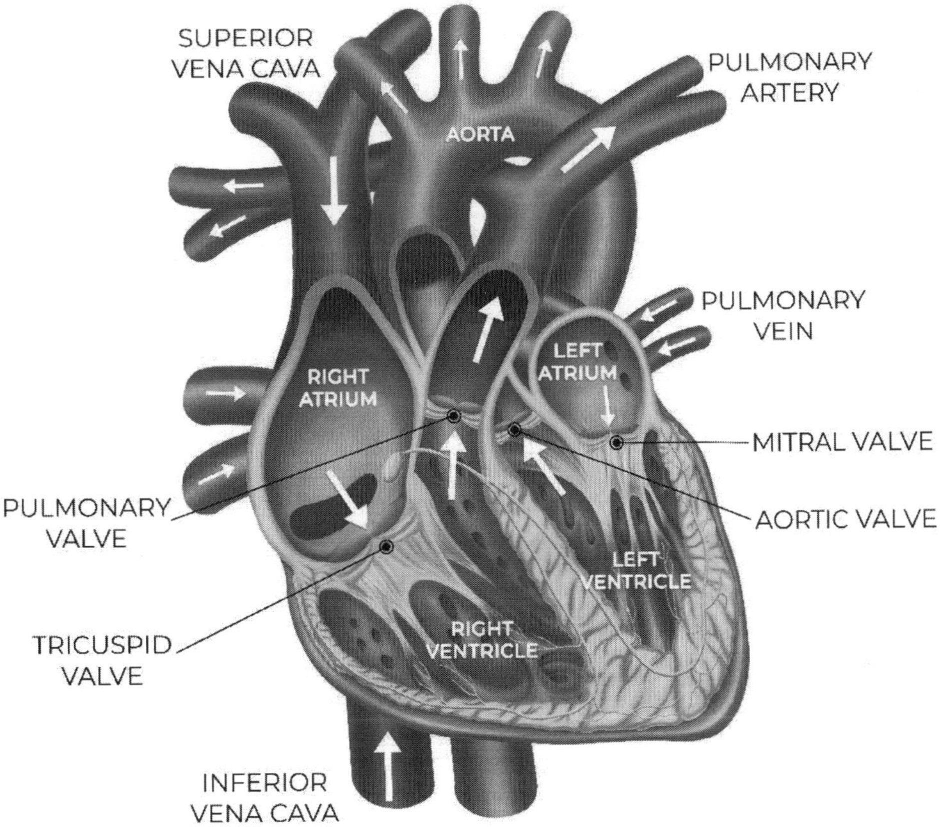

Involvement of Pressure Gradients in Normal Breathing Function

There are four pressures that work together to impact respiratory function. Normal atmospheric pressure at sea level is approximately 760 mm Hg. Atmospheric pressure is important, as pressures inside the body are relative to this number. Intra-alveolar pressure is lower than atmospheric pressure at the beginning of inhalation. This pressure difference assists in drawing air into the lungs in an attempt to equalize pressure. At the beginning of exhalation, intra-alveolar pressure is greater than atmospheric, causing air to passively exit the lungs. At rest, atmospheric pressure is equal to intra-alveolar pressure. Intrapleural pressure is always negative in relation to atmospheric pressure during the normal respiratory cycle. The negative intrapleural pressure exerts a force on the lungs, keeping them close to the chest wall. Finally, transpulmonary pressure is the difference between the intrapleural pressure and the intra-alveolar pressure and is partly responsible for expansion of the lungs during inhalation.

Impact of Resistance and Compliance on the Work of Breathing

Lung compliance is a measurement of how easily the lungs stretch and expand. As lung compliance increases, the work of breathing decreases, since air flows into the lungs more easily. Lung compliance is affected by the elasticity of the lungs, as well by the degree of surface tension. As lung compliance decreases due to disease or injury, the work of breathing increases, as it becomes more difficult to expand the lungs during inspiration. Resistance in the airways refers to how easily air can enter and exit the airways. The biggest contributor to resistance is the diameter of the airway. As airway diameter decreases due to bronchospasms, swelling, or mucus, the resistance to airflow increases. As the issues are alleviated and airway diameter increases and returns to normal, resistance to airflow decreases.

Primary and Secondary Muscles Used for Breathing

Muscles used for breathing are separated into primary and secondary muscle groups. The primary muscle groups are those that are used in normal, quiet breathing. When patients are in respiratory distress and breathing is more difficult, secondary muscle groups become activated. The muscles considered primary for breathing are the diaphragm and the external intercostal muscles. These muscles act by changing the pressure gradient, allowing the lungs to expand and air to flow in and out. The secondary muscle group includes the sternocleidomastoid, scaleni, internal intercostals, obliques, and abdominal muscles. These secondary muscle groups work when breathing is difficult, both in inspiration and expiration, in cases such as obstructions or bronchoconstriction. Use of these secondary muscle groups can often be seen on exam and may be described as see-saw or abdominal breathing (when the abdominal muscles are being used during exhalation) or retractions as the muscles activate and can be seen between rigid structures such as bone.

Features and Landmarks That Should Be Assessed When Interpreting Chest X-Rays

A chest x-ray is one of the quickest diagnostic tests that can be done to evaluate a patient's pulmonary status. It is important to remember when a chest x-ray is performed to assess the entire image and not focus directly on the original reason for the order. Although there are many methods and acronyms people use to remember how to assess a chest x-ray, the same landmarks and features are always assessed. The large airways should be assessed for patency and proper positioning. The bony structures that are visible should be evaluated, including the ribs, clavicles, vertebrae, and any visible appendages. The heart and major vascular structures should be visualized and inspected. The lung fields and pleural spaces should be assessed carefully for any abnormal consolidations, fluid, or air. The diaphragms should be in the correct position. All tubes and lines should also be assessed for proper positioning.

Working of Lungs and Kidneys to Regulate Blood pH

Proper blood pH is critical for correct functioning of all the organs and systems in the body. Blood pH must be maintained within a very narrow range of 7.35 to 7.45, slightly alkalotic. The lungs and the kidneys are the primary organs that regulate this pH balance. The lungs do so by regulating the removal of carbon dioxide from the blood through exhalation. The kidneys do so by regulating the removal of acids and bases depending on which need to be removed. If either of these systems begin to fail, such as respiratory failure, the other system will detect the change in pH level and compensate. For metabolic acidosis, the patient will begin to hyperventilate to bring down the CO_2 levels in the blood, thereby increasing the pH to normal. In metabolic alkalosis, the patient will slow his breathing in order to raise CO_2 levels, thereby lowering the pH. If a respiratory acidosis is present, the kidneys will regulate to lower HCO_3 levels, increasing pH. Finally, if respiratory alkalosis is present, the kidneys will regulate to raise HCO_3 levels, decreasing pH.

Levels of Altered Consciousness

There are six levels of altered consciousness that the respiratory therapist should be aware of when performing an assessment. Understanding these levels can help with assessing whether the patient is able to perform commands or protect his own airway. The six levels are confused, delirious, lethargic, obtunded, stuporous, and comatose. As the patient escalates along these levels, the patient may become more disabled and should be watched closely. Confused patients may or may not be able to perform respiratory therapies, and may need redirecting or reeducation during the therapy. Delirious patients may be unable to follow commands or may even become combative during respiratory therapy. Lethargic patients may easily fall asleep and may not be able to perform prolonged respiratory testing or to complete appropriate MDI administration. Stuporous and comatose patients may have difficulty protecting their own airways and should be evaluated for endotracheal tube placement until underlying neurological issues are resolved.

Characteristics to Note When Assessing the Pulse

When assessing a patient's pulse, it is important to determine more than just the rate. The regularity of the pulse should be assessed to determine if any rhythm irregularities are present. The strength or weakness should be noted. Weak pulses can be indicative of a narrowing pulse pressure (difference between systolic and diastolic pressures) or low cardiac output. Strong or bounding pulses can indicate high blood pressure, decreased elastic ability of the arteries, or increased cardiac output. Pulses should also be assessed at multiple sites to ensure they are easily palpable in all locations and are equal in left and right arteries. An irregular pulse can indicate the presence of an arrhythmia, such as atrial fibrillation, and may require that an EKG be performed. If the pulse is being assessed prior to performing an arterial blood draw, the respiratory therapist should perform an Allen's test.

Various Breathing Patterns and Possible Causes

Kussmaul's respirations are deep, rapid respirations. This type of respiratory pattern is commonly seen in patients who are suffering from a metabolic acidosis, such as diabetic ketoacidosis. Cheyne-Stokes respirations have a crescendo-decrescendo-pause pattern. Patients gradually increase their tidal volume until they take a very large breath and then gradually decrease their tidal volume, followed by a respiratory pause. After the pause, the pattern repeats. This condition is seen in patients following neurological trauma or brain stem injury, as the respiratory center of the brain has been damaged. Biot's respirations involve a very irregular breathing pattern that consists of random respiratory pauses. Unlike Cheyne-Stokes, there is no rhythm or pattern to the respiratory cycle. Biot's is also seen in patients who have suffered a neurological insult to the respiratory center of the brain. Paradoxical breathing is a pattern seen in patients with severe obstructive disease. This pattern is characterized by the abdomen and chest moving in opposite directions during the respiratory cycle. This is commonly seen in children with viral illnesses, such as croup or bronchiolitis, who have trouble exhaling and have increasing CO_2.

Mechanism and Characteristics of Various Breath Sounds

A wheeze is a high-pitched sound that can be heard on inspiration or exhalation. It is caused when air is forced through a restricted airway, such as during bronchospasms or airway edema. The progression of wheezing usually begins with an expiratory wheeze, followed by both inspiratory and expiratory wheezes, and then diminished or absent breath sounds as the airway obstruction becomes more severe. Stridor is also a high-pitched sound, but usually occurs on inspiration and originates in the upper airway, although the sound can be transmitted into the lungs. Coarse breath sounds are low-pitched and are present with fluid, such as in pneumonia or obstructive lung disease. Fine crackles are a result of the small airways being forced open during inspiration and are commonly heard in patients presenting with acute pulmonary edema. Rhonchi can be differentiated from coarse crackles by asking the patient to cough. With rhonchi, the patient should be able to clear the mucus obstruction by coughing.

Important Information to Gather for a Patient's Smoking History

Smoking is a major cause of respiratory disease, including chronic obstructive pulmonary disease, emphysema, lung cancer, and laryngeal cancer. Obtaining the patient's smoking history can help with identifying potential diseases as the patient ages or with diagnosing a new disease with current symptoms. It is important to determine the approximate age the patient began smoking. The younger a person starts smoking, the more damage he can do since the lungs are still developing. The patient's "pack-years" of smoking are determined by how many packs per day for how many years the patient smoked. For example, a patient who has smoked one pack a day for 20 years (20 x 1) and a patient who has smoked 2 packs a day for 10 years (10 x 2) both have a 20 pack-year smoking history. In addition to his own history of smoking, it is important to determine if the patient currently has or has had any past secondhand smoke exposure.

Identifying Features to Note When Evaluating a Neck X-Ray

Neck or upper airway x-rays can be taken for a variety of reasons. Upper airway imaging is commonly performed when diagnosing upper airway obstruction, such as croup, epiglottitis, foreign body obstruction, or tumor invasion. Normally, the trachea should be easily seen as an air-filled column positioned anteriorly in the neck, with a slight narrowing at the vocal cords in the adult. The epiglottis can be visualized near the superior aspect of the trachea and will appear enlarged in a patient with epiglottitis. The nasopharynx and hypopharynx are air-filled cavities that lead from the posterior throat down to the epiglottis. The soft palate can also be identified and evaluated for abnormalities. As with any x-ray, it is important to assess the entire image, noting vertebral, bone, or tissue abnormalities. Focusing only on the airway can cause misidentification of serious disorders.

Clarifying Questions That Can Help Determine Shortness of Breath

When interviewing a patient, it is important to ask questions about the patient's medical history, as well as current medical problems, current medications, allergies, and presenting symptoms to better care for the patient. The patient's medical history should be reviewed to see if he has had any previous respiratory diagnoses or cardiac issues. Specifically, the healthcare provider should ask questions regarding past diagnoses of chronic obstructive pulmonary disease, emphysema, asthma, obstructive sleep apnea, and congestive heart failure. When questioning the patient, be sure to ask the follow questions:

- When did the symptoms begin?
- Was the onset of symptoms sudden or gradual?
- Does anything help to relieve the symptoms?
- What, if anything, makes the symptoms worse?
- Have any medications been taken and did they relieve the symptoms?

Family history should also be reviewed for pulmonary or cardiac conditions.

Monitoring Ventilator Graphics

Ventilator graphics can give a great deal of insight into patient ventilator synchrony. A breath can be divided up into four phases: trigger phase, inspiratory phase, cycle phase, and expiratory phase. By understanding where each of these phases is indicated on a waveform, the clinician can easily identify which is causing patient-ventilator dyssynchrony. In the trigger phase, the most common types of dyssynchrony include auto triggering, double triggering, and missed triggering. Inspiratory phase dyssynchrony can be caused by inappropriate flow rate (too much or too little) or flow pattern. Cycle phase issues involve breath termination, or lack thereof. Expiratory phase issues can be caused by premature exhalation or shortened exhalation time, causing air trapping (auto-PEEP). Ventilator graphics can also distinguish between mechanical, mandatory breaths and patient-triggered breaths.

Factors That Can Elevate Central Venous Pressure/Right Atrial Pressure

Right atrial pressure can be dependent on cardiac output. If blood does not exit the left side of the heart appropriately, it can cause a backup in the system. When the heart is unable to contract efficiently enough to push blood out of the left heart, the blood will not be able to flow into the left side of the heart from the pulmonary vasculature. Pulmonary vascular congestion will follow as blood is unable to push forward. Eventually blood will be unable to leave the right atrium because of the increased pressure, causing distension and pressure elevation in the right atrium. Additionally, pulmonary conditions can increase right heart pressure. Pulmonary hypertension increases resistance and pressure in the pulmonary vasculature, decreasing the amount of blood allowed through. Overdistension of the lungs due to positive pressure ventilation or conditions such as emphysema or asthma can create force on the pulmonary vascular system, increasing pulmonary and right atrial pressures.

Factors That Should Be Assessed When Assessing a Patient's Sputum

A patient's sputum production can give insight into his health. The amount, consistency, color, and even smell of secretions are assessed and can guide practitioners in identifying causes of respiratory infection. The amount of secretions produced increases with pulmonary disease or infection as the body attempts to capture and remove foreign matter. The consistency of sputum also increases as the body fights infection. The thickness of the secretions helps to move foreign material up the mucociliary escalator to be coughed up and out of the body or swallowed and digested. With infections, the color and smell of sputum changes. Yellow or green and foul-smelling sputum are indicators of infection. Pink, frothy sputum can indicate pulmonary edema. Red sputum indicates the presence of blood and can also indicate other pathologies such as cancer.

Basic Neurological Monitoring and Assessment

Neurological disorders can greatly affect the respiratory system if not properly monitored. The degree of neurological monitoring and assessment varies according to the patient's symptoms and medical history. In general, a Glasgow Coma Score (GCS) is an initial assessment done on most patients that assigns a numerical value to the patient's alertness and responsiveness. The highest score is 15 and is assigned to a patient who meets normal assessment criteria. A score of 3 is assigned when a patient has no response to external or painful stimuli. A GCS less than 8 raises concern for severe brain damage, and intubation is usually performed for airway protection. In addition to GCS, it is important to monitor patients for neurological injury that can cause apnea, seizures, or increased intracranial pressure as these conditions can affect the drive to breathe.

Causes of Acute Respiratory Distress in Adult Patients

Respiratory distress in adults can be caused by a number of factors. One of the most common causes is exacerbation of an underlying lung disease, such as Chronic Obstructive Pulmonary Disease (COPD), emphysema, or asthma. Inhalation of irritants (such as smoke), environmental hazards, and occupational hazards can also cause both short-term and long-term respiratory complications. Acute Respiratory Distress Syndrome (ARDS) is a life-threatening disease process that most commonly presents in patients with overwhelming infection (sepsis) or after major bodily trauma, especially thoracic and abdominal trauma. Nonpulmonary causes of respiratory distress include Congestive Heart Failure (CHF), Diabetic Ketoacidosis and renal failure, a distended abdomen, and increased tissue swelling that prevents full movement of the diaphragm and chest cavity. Patients who have had massive blood transfusions are also at high risk for severe respiratory failure.

Characteristics to Assess When Determining Gestational Age of a Newborn

When an infant is born, it is important to determine gestational age, if not known prior to delivery. Gestational age assists in determining care plans and expected outcomes, especially in premature and very premature infants. The most common method of determining gestational age is included in the Ballard Assessment. The Ballard assessment assigns a score for each category assessed. The lower the overall score, the lower the gestational age. Ballard scoring assesses the skin, lanugo (fine hair covering the body), plantar surface (bottom of the foot), breast, eye and ear, and genitals. Possible scores range from -10 (approximately 20 weeks) to 50 (approximately 44 weeks). For every increase of five points, the estimated gestational age increases by two weeks. Ballard scoring should be completed as soon as safely possible once the infant is stable, no more than four days after birth.

Using Palpation to Gather Clinical Data in Respiratory Assessment

Palpation of a patient's chest can be used to elicit a variety of information. Palpation can be used to test for pain or injury to thoracic muscles or bony structures. Chest asymmetry can be detected, indicating pulmonary disorders such as a pneumothorax or flail chest. When hands are placed posteriorly over the diaphragm, an unequal rise in hands can indicate diaphragm muscle disorders and asymmetry. Palpation that reveals crepitus or subcutaneous air can indicate serious respiratory issues in which free air in the thoracic cavity is tracing through subcutaneous tissue. Palpation over the chest during the respiratory cycle, feeling for "crackles" in the chest, can also indicate excess secretions in the large airways. Palpation can also be used to test for vocal fremitus, stronger vibrations that can be felt over abnormally dense areas of lung tissue when a patient speaks.

Mallampati Classification

Mallampati classification refers to a scoring system that rates the ease of intubation. The score ranges from class I to class IV. Class I refers to the ability of the healthcare provider to visualize the airway with no difficulty. Class II refers to a partially obstructed airway in which the healthcare provider can visualize the uvula but not the soft palate of the airway. Class III refers to a partially obstructed airway in which the healthcare provider can visualize only the base of the uvula and not the full uvula or soft palate. Class IV refers to an obstructed airway in which the healthcare provider can visualize none of the soft palate anatomy. The Mallampati classification helps clinicians determine the level of difficulty expected when intubating the patient; for example, a class IV patient may require fiber-optic scopes or other specialized equipment for a successful intubation.

Tracheal Shift

Tracheal shift refers to the displacement of the trachea from the midline to either the left or right side of the chest. A deviated trachea can indicate disorders including but not limited to pneumothorax, pleural effusion, malignant or benign mass presence, and atelectasis. A deviated trachea is often revealed on chest x-rays but can also be seen on visual examination of the chest and neck. Tracheal shift can result in dyspnea, shortness of breath, ventilatory failure, and hypoxia if left untreated. The underlying cause of the tracheal shift must be treated in order to relieve the pressure that forced the trachea to deviate.

Pressure Ulcers as a Result of Respiratory Equipment Use

When using tight-fitting respiratory equipment, skin breakdown can occur. This occurs most frequently when using equipment such as full-face masks, nasal masks, nasal prongs, and other continuous positive airway pressure (CPAP) and bilevel positive airway pressure delivery devices. Pressure ulcers can occur as a result of the extremely tight fit required of these respiratory devices because air leaks in the system can interrupt or decrease airflow to the patient. When using these tight-fitting masks and prongs, it is important to use the lowest level of tightness required to keep the system free of leaks. The skin can also be protected with the use of skin barriers such as DuoDERM and other facility-approved skin protection devices. The respiratory equipment should be changed frequently, and if skin breakdown is noticed, appropriate members of the healthcare team should be notified in order to treat the ulcer before it becomes more severe.

Inspecting a Stoma Site

In patients with a tracheostomy, secretions and pressure on the surrounding airway tissue can cause tissue breakdown and other complications. Therefore, the stoma must be inspected on a regular basis to ensure its patency and general health. The clinician should visually inspect the stoma site for redness or other discoloration, swelling, discharge, odor, and pain. If any of those symptoms occur, report the issue to the appropriate members of the healthcare team for treatment. Lotions should not be applied to the stoma unless directed by the physician. Regular tracheostomy care including inspection, evaluation of patency, and facility-approved cleaning protocols can prevent skin breakdown and help maintain a patent airway.

Pulmonary Artery Size on Chest Radiographs

When viewing a chest radiograph, it is important to note the size of the descending pulmonary arteries. An enlarged right and/or left descending pulmonary artery can indicate pulmonary hypertension. If the right descending pulmonary artery measures more than 16 mm, pulmonary hypertension is possible. Conversely, if the left descending pulmonary artery measures more than 18 mm, pulmonary hypertension is possible. Although the diagnosis of pulmonary hypertension is not based solely on radiograph findings of an enlarged pulmonary artery, the radiograph provides important information that can help the healthcare team make the appropriate diagnosis.

Perform Procedures to Gather Clinical Information

NECESSARY STEPS FOR PERFORMING AN ARTERIAL BLOOD GAS PUNCTURE

As with any procedure, the first step in performing an arterial blood gas is to check for a physician order and ensure that the correct test is being performed on the correct patient. Wash hands and don gloves and any other needed personal protective equipment. Determine whether any extremity is restricted for use (such as a dialysis port or fistula that restricts use of one arm). If a radial site is being used, perform an Allen's test to ensure adequate collateral blood flow to the hand. Sanitize the area with alcohol and carefully insert the needle, using caution not to force it. The needle should be inserted at a 45-degree angle, with the bevel pointing upward. Once blood begins to flow, hold the needle still until the needed amount of blood is collected. Once the sample has been collected, slowly remove the needle and immediately apply pressure to the puncture site with gauze. Pressure may need to be held for up to five minutes to ensure bleeding has stopped. Remove all air from the syringe, remove the needle, and cap the syringe. A patient or lab label should be applied directly to the syringe. If sending to the lab, place the syringe in a cup of ice. The sample should be analyzed as quickly as possible.

DEPOLARIZATION AND REPOLARIZATION IN EKG INTERPRETATION

An EKG (or ECG) is a visual representation of electrical impulses through the heart and is used to assess cardiac rate and rhythm, as well as abnormal variances in heart function in regards to electrical activity. Atrial depolarization is represented on EKG as the P wave. This is the point at which the atria contract and is the first notch on the EKG. The QRS complex is the large spike following the P wave and represents ventricular depolarization. This is where the ventricles contract. The space between the end of the P wave and the beginning of the QRS complex is the PR interval. If the PR interval is too long, it can indicate a delay in conduction between the atria and ventricles. The T wave represents ventricular repolarization and readying of the ventricles for the next heartbeat.

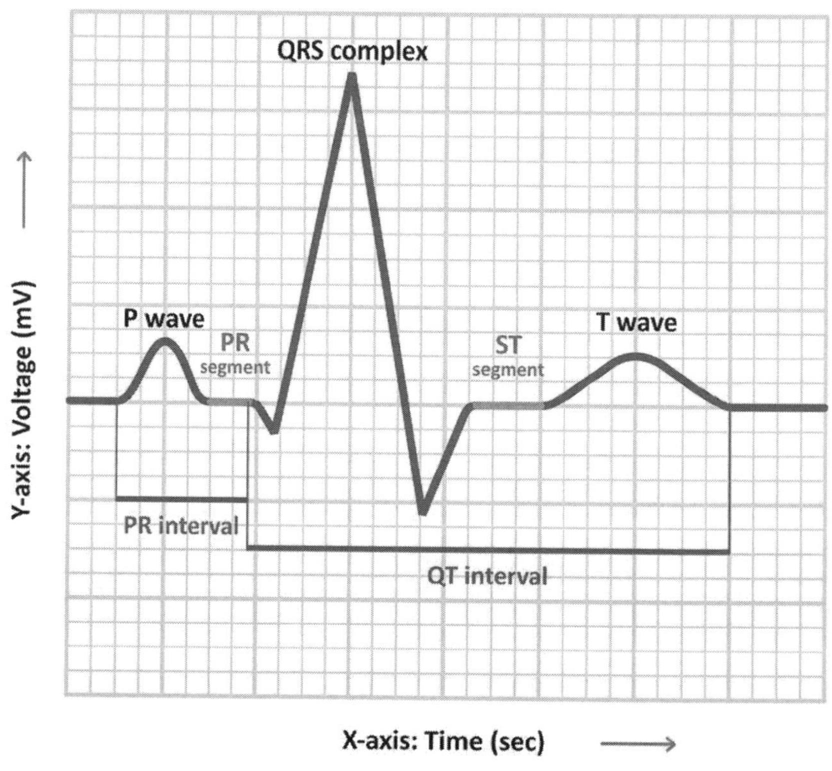

Obtaining a Sputum Culture

Sputum cultures are used to test for bacteria or fungal infections of the lungs. For this reason, obtaining a specimen should be done using a sterile procedure. If the patient is able to cough up sputum on his own, a specimen cup can be placed at the bedside with instructions for the patient to cough any mucus into the cup without touching the inside of the container. Touching the inside of the specimen container can contaminate the specimen and result in a false positive for infection (bacteria may be on the patient's hands, but not in the sputum). If the patient is able to cough, but unable to produce the necessary mucus, a nebulizer with 3% or 7% saline can be used to thin secretions and stimulate removal. If the patient is unable to cough, nasotracheal suctioning can be performed to obtain the sample. For intubated patients, a new, sterile suction catheter should be used for sputum collection. If the patient has an inline suction catheter, it should be replaced with a new one and the sample should be obtained with the first suction attempt. If none of these options are viable, the patient can undergo bronchoscopy to obtain a needed sample. Depending on the reason for obtaining the sample, up to three samples, obtained 8–12 hours apart, may be needed.

Ejection Fraction

Ejection fraction is a measurement that can be obtained by performing an echocardiogram. It measures the percentage of blood that is pumped out of the left ventricle with each ventricular contraction. Normal ejection fraction ranges from 55-65%. This indicates that with each pump of the heart, about 60% of the blood in the left ventricle will be pumped out. Ejection fraction is calculated by dividing the stroke volume (the volume of blood pumped with each beat) by the end-diastolic volume (the volume remaining at the end of the beat) and then multiplying by 100. In patients presenting with heart failure, the stroke volume can rapidly decrease. If the end-diastolic volume remains the same or increases while the stroke volume decreases, the patient's ejection fraction will decrease. Severe heart failure can be diagnosed with an ejection fraction of less than 20%, and is a poor prognostic indicator of future recovery.

Obtaining a Plateau Pressure in an Intubated Patient

Plateau pressure is a measurement of the pressure in the lower airways. Ideal plateau pressure is generally less than 30 cm H_2O to help prevent lung damage from barotrauma (damage caused by pressure) and overdistension of lung tissue. Plateau pressure, in addition to Peak Inspiratory Pressure, are useful tools in determining the patient's current level of lung disease, such as an increased airway resistance or a decrease in pulmonary compliance. For an intubated patient, plateau pressures can be measured by performing an end inspiratory hold on the ventilator. It is important to remember that plateau pressures are not static and can change quickly. For this reason, plateau pressures should be monitored and documented frequently for early identification of compliance changes. To minimize plateau pressures in intubated patients, smaller tidal volumes may need to be used, especially for patients with Acute Respiratory Distress Syndrome.

Measuring the Rapid Shallow Breathing Index (RSBI)

The Rapid Shallowing Breathing Index is a calculation used for intubated patients when assessing the patient's readiness to extubate. The RSBI is obtained by multiplying the patient's respiratory rate by the tidal volume. In general, the higher the calculated RSBI, the less likely a patient is to tolerate spontaneous breathing and extubation. This high result is usually related to a patient who is breathing too quickly and shallowly. Patients will be unable to continue this pattern for any extended period of time before succumbing to fatigue and respiratory failure. An RSBI of less than 105 breaths/min/L is generally considered "passing" and is associated with better outcomes once the patient has been extubated.

Tests to Assess Respiratory Muscle Strength

The two most common tests performed to assess a patient's respiratory muscle strength are the Negative Inspiratory Force (NIF) and the Vital Capacity (VC) maneuvers. These measurements can be obtained for intubated or extubated patients. Assessing a patient's muscle strength is most commonly done prior to extubation to ensure that the patient has the strength to breathe once the endotracheal tube is removed. Assessment is also performed on patients who present with progressive neuromuscular disease, such as myasthenia gravis or Guillain-Barré, as a way to keep ahead of potential respiratory failure. The NIF and VC maneuvers are tools that are commonly performed together and can be used to trend a patient's status. If both numbers are decreasing, it indicates a decrease in the patient's ability to take a deep breath, and eventually the patient may become too weak to keep a normal pH and will develop a respiratory acidosis.

CVP, PAP, and PCWP

Central Venous Pressure (CVP) is a measurement used to estimate the pressure in the right atrium. This measurement can be used to assess preload and fluid status and determine whether there is evidence of right-sided heart failure. CVP pressures can be measured with the use of a central venous catheter (cm H_2O) or a Swan-Ganz catheter (mm Hg). A normal CVP pressure is 8 cm H_2O or less or 6 mm Hg or less. Pulmonary Artery Pressure (PAP) is measured with a Swan-Ganz catheter in the pulmonary artery. It is used to estimate left ventricular preload and is normally between 20 and 30 mm Hg. Pulmonary Capillary Wedge Pressure (PCWP) is also measured with a Swan-Ganz catheter and is used to estimate the left atrial pressure. Normal range is between 4 and 12 mm Hg.

Obtaining Endotracheal Cuff Pressures

There are three common methods for verifying appropriate cuff pressure in an endotracheal or tracheostomy tube. When possible, the desired method is to use a pressure manometer to determine exact pressure within the cuff. Ideally, cuff pressures should be kept less than 25 cm H_2O to keep minimal pressure from exertion on the tracheal wall. If a pressure manometer is unavailable, a minimal leak technique can be performed by slowly drawing air out of the cuff until a small leak is heard. Another method is the minimal occlusion technique: after performing the minimal leak test, enough air is reinserted to occlude the leak. The minimal occlusion technique is recommended above the minimal leak technique to decrease the risk of aspiration that can lead to ventilator-associated pneumonia. These methods ensure that the pressure being exerted on the trachea is only the minimum needed for ventilation. Checking cuff pressures frequently and documenting them is the best way to prevent tracheal damage.

Monitoring Renal Function in Critically Ill Patients

Since the kidneys play a critical role, along with the cardiopulmonary system, in maintaining proper blood pH, monitoring the level of injury is an important part of the respiratory therapist's assessment. One of the major marks of renal function is the ability to produce an appropriate level of urine. If urine production decreases, the patient can quickly become unstable as fluid and toxins build up in the body. Blood work is also analyzed to determine renal function. Glomerular filtration rate (GFR) can be used to monitor or diagnose acute kidney injury or failure. On average, normal GFR ranges from 90 to 120 mL/min/1.73m^2, with renal injury diagnosed for GFR below 60 mL/min/1.73m^2. In some cases, clinicians can become so concerned that they might give too much fluid that the patient does not receive enough. Proper fluid balance and adequate blood pressure are two important measurements to watch closely in the beginning of an acute illness. Impaired renal function in acutely ill patients has been shown to increase morbidity and mortality.

Nutritional Monitoring in Critically Ill Patients

A patient's nutritional status can greatly impact their ability to heal after illness and their length of recovery. Proper nutrition is needed when a patient is critically ill to maintain overall health status and organ function. Nutritional status can be evaluated with blood work and by monitoring the patient's intake and output measurements. Inappropriate nutrition can lead to increased days on ventilator, longer intensive care unit stay, and longer hospital stays. Without proper nutrition, muscle atrophy can happen at an accelerated rate, including the muscles used for breathing. Wound healing and infection clearing can also take longer without adequate nutrition. A clinical nutritionist who specializes in acute and critical care patients can be a great resource for managing a patient's nutritional intake. In particular, the amount of protein should be calculated based on the patient's needs. A patient with chronic respiratory disorders, such as COPD, also needs close monitoring of carbohydrates, as they break down in the body and can increase CO_2 levels.

Possible Causes of Ventilator Dependence

Timely weaning from mechanical ventilation in the intensive care unit is a key role of the respiratory therapist. Ventilator dependence can be caused by a variety of processes, both respiratory and nonrespiratory in origin. Patients with prolonged intubation due to critical illness can become ventilator dependent due to muscle atrophy and muscle fatigue. Patients with underlying disease processes, such as COPD, can be ventilator dependent as the disease progresses. Neuromuscular disorders that cause a progressive decrease in muscle tone and strength can also cause dependence, as the patient will no longer be able to use his respiratory muscles. In addition, damage or insult to the respiratory center of the brain can cause frequent apnea in patients, requiring ventilator dependence. Tracheostomy should be considered to aid in the weaning process if it is determined that the patient will have a prolonged ventilator course.

Assessing a Patient's Readiness for Liberation from the Ventilator

Patients who are being assessed for their ability to breathe without the ventilator must prove that they are ready to do so. The patient should be placed in a spontaneous breathing mode to determine whether he has the drive to breathe. If there is no internal drive to breathe, the rest of the exam is futile. Muscle strength to breathe can be assessed with a spontaneous breathing trial in pressure support mode or through a T-piece trial. Multiple spontaneous breathing trials may be needed to help build muscle strength and stamina. The patient should also be able to demonstrate protection of the airway with an intact cough and gag reflex. Ideally, the patient should be able to answer simple yes or no questions, but if all other criteria are met, the ability to follow commands is not necessary for a trial of extubation.

Issues Affecting a Patient's Ability to Wean from Mechanical Ventilation

Almost every other organ system in the body can have an effect on a patient's ability to wean from mechanical ventilation. The neurological system can affect a patient's drive to breathe, as well as his ability to breathe, based on nerve innervation and muscle strength. If the cardiovascular system is failing, the patient may become fluid overloaded, causing pulmonary edema. Heart failure can also increase respiratory distress as the respiratory system attempts to compensate for the failing heart and decreased tissue oxygenation. If the renal system is injured, the kidneys will not be able to remove toxins and fluid from the body. In addition, the renal system plays an important role in balancing blood pH, and kidney disease can alter this balance. If the renal system is unable to regulate bicarbonate, the respiratory system will compensate, causing either tachypnea or bradypnea.

Psychological and Physiological Factors That Should Be Addressed Prior to Extubation

Every attempt should be made to optimize the patient prior to extubation. Intubation can create psychological issues for patients when they are awake, but consciousness is necessary for extubation. It can be helpful to talk to the patient, telling him exactly what to expect and alleviating some of the discomfort and anxiety of the unknown. Anti-anxiety medication can help the patient through the extubation process with minimal sedative side effects. Physiologically, the patient should have stable vital signs, including heart rate, oxygen saturation, and blood pressure. The patient should not have excess fluid. Fluid can be measured by monitoring the patient's intake and output or by weighing the patient and comparing with the admission weight. Any infections should be treated, or should currently be in treatment, with limited chance of compromising the airway. The patient should not have any major surgeries planned in the near future that would require re-intubation.

Performing a Spontaneous Breathing Trial

Prior to performing a spontaneous breathing trial, the patient should have sedation stopped or minimized to prevent medication-related apneic events. The patient should be awake and instructed that the trial is about to begin. Minimal sedation should be used only if the patient is uncooperative or at risk for self-harm by removing medical devices. A full assessment should be performed, including breath sounds, heart rate, respiratory rate, oxygen saturation, and end tidal CO_2 readings. Once it is determined that the patient is stable enough for a trial, he can be switched to a spontaneous breathing mode. After transitioning modes, the tidal volumes, minute ventilation, peak pressures, and vital signs should all be noted so that any changes during the trial can be identified. The length of the breathing trial can vary by institution, but usually ranges from 30 minutes to 2 hours. At the end of the trial, a full assessment should be repeated to ensure the patient tolerated the trial well. An arterial blood gas can be drawn if there is any concern over how the patient handled the trial. At the end of the trial, the patient can be placed back on the previous settings or extubated. Spontaneous breathing trials can be performed daily if needed to keep the patient's inspiratory muscles from weakening, but should always be performed prior to an extubation.

Performing Peak Flow and Interpreting Results at Home

A peak flow meter is a device that measures the maximum flow a patient can produce on exhalation. Many patients with asthma use it on a daily basis to predict asthma attacks early. In many cases, a decreasing peak flow can be an initial indicator that lung function is decreasing and resistance is increasing, even prior to noticeable symptoms. A peak flow should be performed at the same time every day. The time of day is less important than the consistency of the timing. The patient should be in an upright position to allow for full lung inflation. When ready, the patient should fully exhale, followed by a full inhale. Lips should be wrapped fully around the mouthpiece. The patient should exhale as quickly and forcefully as possible into the peak flow meter and the result should be logged. Up to three attempts can be made with a rest period between each. The patient is in the "green zone" when he is able to produce peak flow measurements of 80–100% of their baseline value. If the patient measures between 50–80% of baseline value, he is in the "yellow zone" and should monitor symptoms closely and begin to take additional medications as instructed by a physician. Under 50% of baseline is considered the "red zone" and the patient should seek care from a physician or emergency room as indicated in his asthma action plan.

Important Information to Obtain Before Preparing for an Arterial Puncture

An arterial puncture is a common procedure done by respiratory therapists, especially in the intensive care units and the emergency department. Although routine, consequences can be severe if it is not performed correctly. Prior to a radial arterial puncture, an Allen's test or modified Allen's test should be performed to ensure that the patient has adequate collateral circulation with the ulnar artery in the event that the radial artery sustains damage during the puncture. If the Allen's test is negative, it should be documented and another site should be identified. The patient's chart should also be reviewed to assess for limb limitations, especially in regards to implantation of shunts for dialysis. Finally, information regarding the patient's coagulation status should be obtained, including platelet count and whether the patient is on anticoagulation therapy, such as heparin.

Factors Affecting Accurate Readings When Performing Pulse Oximetry

When assessing the accuracy of a pulse oximetry, it is important to determine the validity of the data. Many factors can interfere with a pulse oximetry reading and incorrect reading can greatly affect the patient care plan. Patient perfusion can have a big impact on how well the pulse oximeter is reading. Patients with low peripheral perfusion may have inaccurate readings, as the sensors are unable to accurately read the saturated hemoglobin levels when there is not enough blood present. Warming the extremity can help increase perfusion and give a more accurate reading. Patient movement is another common cause of inaccurate readings. When possible, the extremity with the pulse oximeter on it should be immobile before recording the reading. Fluorescent lights can cause lower readings, so when troubleshooting the pulse oximeter, it may be helpful to cover the extremity with a blanket to block extra light.

Performing Spontaneous Breathing Trials

A spontaneous breathing trial is best performed during normal waking hours, typically in the morning. This allows the patient to be as awake as possible. Spontaneous breathing trials are usually performed in one of two ways. The first way is to place the patient on a spontaneous mode of ventilation, such as pressure support or volume support. The patient can then breathe at his own rate but is still connected to the ventilator in case he becomes apneic or needs additional support. The second method is the T-piece trial. In this method, the patient is removed from the ventilator completely and a T-piece is connected to the end of the endotracheal tube with oxygen attached. This method tests muscle strength, as the patient must do all the work with no assistance. In either method, the spontaneous breathing trial usually lasts anywhere from 30 minutes to 2 hours. At the end of the trial, the patient is assessed to determine whether extubation is feasible. If not, the patient will be returned to the ventilator.

Role of Continuous Overnight Pulse Oximetry in Diagnosing Sleep Disorders

Continuous overnight pulse oximetry can be used for patients in lieu of, or prior to, a sleep study. In most cases, an overnight sleep study is performed while a patient is admitted to the hospital. A pulse oximeter is attached to the patient with a machine that records the patient's vital signs, including heart rate and SpO_2. The data is then uploaded and analyzed. The number of desaturations below a certain level is documented and can be used to determine whether the patient would benefit from nocturnal oxygen or the initiation of CPAP therapy. In most cases, insurance requires a full sleep study before covering CPAP, but an overnight pulse oximetry study is a quick, painless screening tool to determine whether a full sleep study is indicated.

Determining Auto-PEEP in Intubated Patients

Auto-PEEP occurs when the patient's expiratory time is insufficient. When a patient is intubated, auto-PEEP can be caused by several factors, both by the patient (increased expiratory airway resistance) and by the practitioner (inappropriate ventilator settings). Detecting auto-PEEP can be done several ways. An end-expiratory hold can be completed, which closes the exhalation valve at the end of exhalation. This will detect total airway PEEP, and if it is greater than the set value, the patient has auto-PEEP. Analyzing the pressure waveform can also indicate auto-PEEP if the waveform fails to return to baseline before the next breath is initiated. Analyzing volumes can also indicate auto-PEEP if volume returned is less than volume set or if the volume waveform does not return to baseline before the next breath is initiated. Finally, if flow is present through the entire expiratory phase, and the patient is not using accessory expiratory muscles to forcefully exhale, this can indicate auto-PEEP. Flow should return to zero before the next breath is initiated.

Titrating CPAP Levels to Determine Appropriate Levels in Sleep Apnea Patients

When a patient presents for a sleep study, the patient will typically be observed for a full night. After this, the study will be reviewed by a sleep specialist and the patient will return for another sleep study with CPAP applied. The technician will apply the CPAP and the patient will be observed during sleep to see if the level of CPAP is sufficient. If the patient still has multiple apnea/desaturation events, the technician will titrate the CPAP level up until the events are below the set threshold. If the patient presents for the initial sleep study and after a few hours his condition is deemed to be severe, the technician can wake the patient up and apply CPAP that night, titrating as needed until the morning. In mild cases, the patient may be given a beginning CPAP level and sent home to use the machine. The CPAP level will be titrated based on the patient's subjective symptoms. Some newer CPAP machines have the ability to titrate to the patient's need once a lower and upper limit have been set.

Using Transcutaneous Blood Gas Monitoring in the Critically Ill

Transcutaneous blood gas monitoring allows providers to trend the patient's arterial CO_2 and O_2 without frequently drawing blood from the patient. This is especially useful in patients who are severely ill and in need of frequent blood gases to make ventilator changes. Although transcutaneous monitoring is not as exact as arterial blood gases, it does allow the clinician to observe whether the patient's CO_2 and O_2 are trending in the desired direction or whether additional ventilator changes need to be made. Transcutaneous monitoring is popular in the neonatal population, but it is becoming more common in adult patients as well. For adults, the monitoring probe needs to be placed on an area with a thinner cutaneous layer, such as the earlobe, to get the most precise reading.

Apnea Test (Brain Death Determination)

Purpose of an Apnea Test

When determining brain death, clinicians use an apnea test as one of several deciding factors. The apnea test is a mandatory evaluation that helps to determine the absence of brain stem activity. Absence of brain activity is one factor in the determination of brain death; therefore, apnea testing is a mandatory evaluation for patients who are presumed to be brain dead. Apnea testing is associated with complications including but not limited to hypoxia, hypotension, pneumothorax, hypercarbia, cardiac arrhythmias, and asystole. To minimize these risks, clinicians follow their facility-approved apnea testing protocol to properly prepare the patient for testing and ensure the patient's safety and comfort during the procedure.

Procedure of an Apnea Test

When performing an apnea test, the patient must be properly prepared in order to minimize any adverse events associated with testing. First, the body temperature needs to be a minimum of 32 degrees Celsius. This helps to ensure stable hemodynamics during the procedure. Next, the patient should be preoxygenated if needed in order to maintain PaO_2 levels and minimize the risk of hypoxia during the test. The patient should also have a stable fluid balance and stable blood pressure with a systolic value of 90 mm Hg or more. The apnea test is then conducted by either disconnecting the patient from the ventilator or by turning the ventilator mode to a spontaneous mode. The patient is observed for the presence of respiration. If no respiration occurs at a $PaCO_2$ of 60 mm Hg (or 20 mm Hg from the patient's baseline), then the patient is considered to be apneic and the procedure confirms brain death.

Tests of Respiratory Muscle Strength — MIP and MEP

Maximal inspiratory pressure (MIP) testing is an evaluation of a patient's inspiratory muscle strength, although maximal expiratory pressure (MEP) testing is an evaluation of a patient's expiratory muscle strength. These are important tests for determining extubation readiness because the patient must have adequate respiratory muscle strength in order to be successfully extubated and take over the work of breathing without ventilatory support. Prior to extubation, the patient will undergo MIP and MEP testing. During these bedside tests, the patient inhales against a closed circuit with an attached manometer (MIP test) and exhales against a similar circuit (MEP test). The MIP test measures the MIP that the patient can achieve. This test is also often referred to as a negative inspiratory force (NIF) test, because the manometer is measuring the maximum negative force that the patient can achieve when inhaling.

Evaluate Procedure Results

Components of Total Lung Capacity (TLC)

Total lung capacity is determined by having a patient complete a pulmonary function test (PFT). Total lung capacity is defined as the amount of air in the lungs after a person takes the largest inhalation possible. In regards to testing, total lung capacity can be divided into four components. The individual components that are abnormal assist in diagnosis of lung disease and help to direct treatment. *Tidal volume* is the amount of air inspired during a normal breath. The maximum amount of air that is forcefully inspired above normal tidal volume is considered the *inspiratory reserve volume*. The maximum amount of air that can be forcefully exhaled after a normal exhalation is considered the *expiratory reserve volume*. *Residual volume* is the amount of air left in the lungs after a maximum exhalation. Total lung capacity is the combination of all four of these measurements.

Role of a Sputum Gram Stain and Culture in Pulmonary Diagnosis

A sputum gram stain and culture is a microbiology test of a patient's sputum to identify the pathological cause of a respiratory infection. Determining the exact nature of the infection is important for treating the disease, as well as preventing its spread by instituting the correct isolation precautions. Depending on what the gram stain and culture reveal about the infection, the patient may need to be placed on droplet or airborne isolation precautions to protect healthcare workers, as well as other patients and the patient's own family and friends. In some instances, test results may place a restriction on visitors until the infection is treated. From a treatment perspective, the test results may change the current course of treatment to more specific medications, such as stronger, narrow spectrum antibiotics or antifungals, or even inhaled antibiotics.

Reasons for Performing a Pulmonary Function Test

The most common reason for performing a pulmonary function test is to assess for or monitor a pulmonary impairment, such as COPD, asthma, pulmonary fibrosis, cystic fibrosis, etc. Chronic respiratory diseases worsen over time, so frequent surveillance with a pulmonary function test helps to identify declining lung function early. In addition, pulmonary function tests can be performed for the following reasons:

1. To provide surveillance on healthy people in the general population to help identify normal values,
2. To determine preoperatively whether the patient has an increased risk of pulmonary complications in the postoperative recovery phase,
3. To determine whether current medications or interventions are increasing pulmonary function,
4. To quantify the degree of disability for insurance or work purposes, and
5. To determine transplant eligibility and postoperative risk level for patients seeking lung or heart transplants.

Determining Restrictive Lung Disease and Obstructive Lung Disease with Pulmonary Function Tests

Pulmonary function tests can be used to determine whether a patient has a restrictive or obstructive process, as these are treated differently but have overlapping symptoms. In an obstructive process, determining the patient's flow measurements will reveal decreases in forced vital capacity (FVC), forced expiratory volume in 1 second (FEV1), forced expiratory volume/forced vital capacity (FEV/FVC), and forced expiratory flow (FEF) values. These changes represent an increase in airway resistance. In contrast, restrictive lung disease is a decrease in pulmonary compliance and will have an impact on lung volumes and capacities. On a pulmonary function test, the values related to volumes, such as inspiratory reserve volume (IRV), expiratory reserve volume (ERV), residual volume (RV), and functional residual capacity (FRC), will all be decreased. Some patients can present with both obstructive and restrictive components of lung disease, and therefore may have decreases in all of the above values.

Effect of Body Temperature on Arterial Blood Gas Results

Normal values listed for arterial blood gas results assume the patient is normothermic (37°C). When patients are hypothermic or hyperthermic, corrections must be made to obtain the correct value. Most blood gas analyzers will ask for the patient's temperature when analyzing so that corrected measurements can be reported. Patients who are hypothermic tend to have decreased PCO_2 and PO_2 due to an increase in gas solubility. This subsequently leads to an increase in the pH value (alkalosis). Hyperthermic patients have higher PCO_2 and PO_2 due to a decrease in gas solubility, leading to a decrease in pH (acidosis). Additionally, body temperature changes can shift the O_2 dissociation curve to the left (hypothermia) or to the right (hyperthermia), affecting the availability of oxygen to the tissues.

Interpreting Sleep Study Results

Sleep study results should be interpreted by a physician trained in sleep medicine, usually a neurologist or pulmonologist since the results can impact a patient's qualification for home therapy, such as CPAP devices, and insurance coverage of services. A sleep study monitors vital signs, such as heart rate, respiratory rate, and oxygen levels, as well as brain waves, to detect sleep stages and flow impedance at the airway openings. The number of desaturations per hour has a major impact on the outcome of a sleep study, along with the number of apneas. The number of times a patient wakes and sleep stage disturbance is also analyzed. The apnea-hypopnea index is also used, which analyzes the number of apnea events and the number of hypopnea events per hour. An apnea-hypopnea index of five or less is considered normal, while 30 or higher is considered severe sleep apnea.

First-Degree, Second-Degree Type I and II, and Third-Degree Heart Blocks

First-degree heart block is a slowing of the signal between the atrium and ventricle. This produces an abnormally long PR interval on EKG. This type of heart block is not an emergency, and many times the patient has no symptoms. Second-degree heart block is also a slowing of the signal between the atrium and ventricle, but on a larger scale. There are two types of second-degree heart block: type I and type II. Type I (also known as Wenckebach) occurs when the signal between the atrium and ventricle becomes more and more delayed with each beat until a QRS complex "drops," and the signal does not progress through the ventricle at all. The patient may complain of occasional dizziness or lightheadedness with this arrhythmia. Type II is more severe and occurs when some signals progress to the ventricles and others do not. It is less rhythmic than Type I. In many cases, the patient will need a pacemaker placed to assist the ventricle in contracting when the signal does not progress from the atrium. Third-degree heart block occurs when none of the signals from the atrium reach the ventricles. It is also known as complete heart block. In a third-degree block, the heart's backup system may kick in and the patient will present with bradycardia with extra P-waves on EKG. Third-degree heart block can be life threatening and a pacemaker is necessary.

Interpreting Six-Minute Walk Test Results

A six-minute walk test is performed as part of an assessment for patients with a variety of cardiopulmonary diseases. In cardiac or pulmonary rehabilitation programs, patients complete a six-minute walk test in the beginning, at set intervals during, and at the end of the program to assess their endurance. The test assesses not only how far the patient is able to walk in six minutes, but the subjective level of dyspnea, the heart rate, and the oxygenation level. As the patient progresses through a rehabilitation program, he should show improvement by completing a greater distance in six minutes, with less dyspnea. Six-minute walk tests are often completed as part of a transplant program for heart and lung transplants to make sure the patient remains a good candidate for a transplant.

Review Video: How Does the Six Minute Walk Test Work?
Visit mometrix.com/academy and enter code: 444929

Blood Gas Results in Newborns vs. Adults

During the birthing process, there are major transitions that occur in the cardiopulmonary system. As the fetus passes through the birth canal, compression of the umbilical cord diminishes flow from the placenta to the fetus. Since gas and nutrient exchange happens in the placenta, this compression decreases gas exchange for the fetus. Once the baby is delivered and the cord is clamped, the newborn is stimulated to breathe several ways, including external stimulation in the new environment and internal stimulation through changes in pH and CO_2 levels. Since newborns need to generate a great amount of pressure (up to 60 cm H_2O) to open the lungs for the initial breath, it takes time for the newborn to compensate. Therefore, if a blood gas is drawn on a newborn, the normal pH will be acidotic (7.30–7.35) and the CO_2 will be increased (50 mm Hg). Additionally, the patient will be hypoxemic, with PaO_2 of 20–30 mm Hg.

Waveform Analysis When Evaluating Capnography

Capnography is the continuous monitoring of a patient's end tidal carbon dioxide. It can be used on patients via noninvasive and invasive means. When connected to a monitor, the capnography gives both a number (exhaled CO_2) and a waveform. When assessing the waveform, a variety of aspects should be monitored. The height of the waveform correlates with the value of the exhaled CO_2. As CO_2 increases, the height of the waveform also increases. The rhythm correlates with the respiratory pattern. If the patient is breathing consistently, the rhythm will also be consistent. Inspiratory pauses or abnormal patterns, such as Cheyne-Stokes, will be seen on the end tidal waveform. In conjunction with rhythm, the frequency of breaths can be assessed. A patient's respiratory rate should correlate with the frequency of the waveform.

Explaining Peak Flow Meter Results to Patients

A peak flow meter is used to measure and monitor a patient's airway resistance to expiratory flow, especially in asthma patients. As a patient's airway resistance increases, such as with inflammation or bronchoconstriction, the peak expiratory flow will decrease. Patients should be performing a peak flow maneuver on a daily basis, ideally at the same time of day, to evaluate lung function. In many cases, a declining peak flow value can be the initial sign of an impending asthma attack. Patients are instructed on the "red," "yellow," and "green" zones of the peak flow. When patients are able to achieve 80% to 100% of their best peak flow value, they are considered to be in the green zone and should continue with their current regimen. When the peak flow is between 50% and 80% of the patient's best value, the patient is considered to be in the yellow zone. Less than 50% of their best value is considered the red zone and indicates an asthma attack. For each zone, the patient should have a prescribed therapy to follow, including scheduled short-acting bronchodilators, when to call the physician for additional recommendations, and when to visit the emergency room.

Screening Spirometry in a Patient's Surgical Workup

For patients with pre-existing pulmonary conditions, such as COPD, it may be beneficial to screen patients prior to any non-emergent surgery. Patients with lung issues may be at a higher risk of postoperative problems, including difficulty weaning from the ventilator, pneumonia, increased hospital length of stay, and increased morbidity and mortality. Spirometry is a quick, inexpensive test that can be performed for high-risk patients, allowing the pulmonologist to gauge the risk level. Those who perform well on the preoperative spirometry screening are considered lower risk. If a patient performs poorly, he is considered higher risk. For high-risk patients, the risk versus benefit of the surgery, especially if it is an elective surgery, must be weighed carefully and alternative medical management may be required instead of surgery.

Negative Inspiratory Force and Vital Capacity Measurements

Neuromuscular diseases, such as Guillain-Barré, myasthenia gravis, or multiple sclerosis, cause progressive weakness. Each disease affects the body differently, but all have the risk of causing weakened respiratory muscles, leading to respiratory failure. Negative Inspiratory Force (NIF) measures the strength of a patient's inspiratory muscles. When performed routinely in the hospital, it can give care providers an idea of muscle strength and indicate whether the disease is progressing or improving. As muscle strength is impacted, the NIF measurement will become less negative (closer to zero), while large negative numbers (-60) equate to greater strength. Vital capacity (VC) measures the volume the patient can exhale with maximal effort. Again, as muscle strength weakens, the amount becomes smaller. Larger volumes are equated with increased muscle strength. NIF and VC are best used as trending tools, rather than an individual or one-time assessment.

Effects of Preload and Afterload on Blood Pressure

Preload is the pressure needed to fill the heart at the end of diastole (heart muscle relaxation). Preload is measured by the pressure in the left atrium at the end of diastole. As preload increases, the volume in the heart at the end of diastole will also increase. If preload becomes insufficient, the heart will not be able to pump enough blood, lowering blood pressure. Afterload is the pressure the heart must pump against to get blood out of the left ventricle during systole. When afterload is low, the heart's work is also lessened, allowing blood to easily leave the heart during contraction. As afterload increases, the heart's work also increases, decreasing the amount of blood leaving the left ventricle with each beat (stroke volume).

Scenarios

An EKG is performed on a patient and it is noted the patient is in atrial fibrillation. Discuss concerns associated with this rhythm.

> Atrial fibrillation is a quivering of the atrium without any true contraction. It can be caused by an ectopic area of the atrium sending out impulses. In cases of atrial fibrillation, the AV node will determine the rate of ventricle contraction. Atrial fibrillation can be a very worrisome rhythm when left untreated. Atrial fibrillation with rapid ventricular response (RVR) can cause the heart to beat at extremely high levels, decreasing perfusion and oxygen delivery and lowering a patient's blood pressure since the heart is cannot fill with blood while beating so fast. During normal rhythms, the ventricles rely on the "atrial kick" to help fill them during atrial contraction. In atrial fibrillation, this kick is absent, causing inadequate filling of the ventricles. Finally, because the atrium does not fully contract, blood can become stagnant in the atrium, placing the patient at a higher risk of blood clots and pulmonary embolism.

A patient with advanced emphysema shows increased functional residual capacity and reserve volume, as well as a decrease in vital capacity, on a PFT. Explain the physiological reasoning behind these results.

> Emphysema is a chronic, irreversible, obstructive lung disease. It is characterized by destruction of the alveolar wall, creating larger terminal airway sacs. This alveolar destruction decreases the surface area available for gas exchange, making it more difficult to exchange oxygen and carbon dioxide. Additionally, the obstructive component decreases the ability to exhale, trapping air in the distal airways. This increases the functional residual capacity and reserve volume. The more that emphysema makes changes to the lung tissue, the greater these volumes will be on a pulmonary function test. FVC and FVC1 will be decreased due to the obstruction and the increase in expiratory airway resistance. As emphysema continues to advance, the lungs can become so overdistended that even small breaths will become extremely difficult.

Distinguishing Between Obstructive and Restrictive Lung Disease Using FEV1 and FVC

In both obstructive and restrictive lung disease, FVC and FEV1 can be below the expected value, but the reason for the decreased values is different for each type of disease. In restrictive diseases, the patient has difficulty inhaling due to airway restriction, and all lung volumes will be lower than expected. In obstructive diseases, exhalation is obstructive and air trapping occurs. To distinguish between obstructive lung disease and restrictive lung disease based on the FEV1 and the FVC, the FEV1/FVC ratio needs to be examined. In the obstructive lung disease patient, the FEV1/FVC ratio will be less than 70% of the FVC due to obstruction during exhalation. In restrictive lung patients, the ratio will be greater than 70% as the patient is unable to inhale a large breath, meaning inhalation and exhalation are nearly equal.

Evaluating Cuff Pressure/Volume

When assessing the cuff pressure of a patient's airway, the standard should be to measure with a cuff manometer. The cuff manometer measures cuff pressures via the pilot balloon. Appropriate cuff pressures of 20–30 cm H_2O help to create a seal within the airway without overdistending and increasing risk of airway damage. Appropriate cuff pressures help to minimize aspiration risk and prevent ventilator-associated pneumonias and infections. If a cuff manometer is unavailable, minimal occlusion volume (MOV) is the next best technique. For MOV, air is slowly inserted into the cuff until there is no air leakage. This should be repeated at set intervals, 2–3 times daily, to ensure that only the minimum needed amount of air is used. Minimal leak technique (MLT) should be avoided as this leaves enough of a leak for aspiration, increasing the possibility of pneumonia.

Evaluating Obstructive Sleep Apnea Using Overnight Pulse Oximetry

Overnight pulse oximetry is used either in place of or prior to a complete sleep study when a patient is suspected of having obstructive sleep apnea. It is performed with a pulse oximetry monitor that saves the information so that it can be downloaded and interpreted after the study is completed. If the patient has numerous, sustained desaturation episodes throughout the night, this is an indicator that the patient has obstructive sleep apnea. When the desaturation events are significant enough, obstructive sleep apnea therapy, such as CPAP therapy, may be initiated and the pulse oximetry study may be repeated with the CPAP device in place. An overnight pulse oximetry study is inexpensive and easy, unlike a sleep study in which heart, breathing, and EEG leads all need to be placed.

Evaluating Spontaneous Breathing Trial Results for Discontinuation of Mechanical Ventilation

Results of a spontaneous breathing trial are evaluated to determine if a patient can be disconnected from mechanical ventilation. Spontaneous breathing trials performed in preparation for extubation generally last about two hours, but the time limit may vary depending on the specific institution's policy. After two hours, or the completion of the trial, if the patient meets the criteria, and any additional requirements, he has an increased chance of successful extubation. The normal criteria include: a total respiratory rate of less than 30 breaths per minute, a PaO_2/FiO_2 ratio of greater than 150 with a PEEP of 5–8 or less and an FiO_2 of 0.4–0.5 or less, and hemodynamic stability. The patient should also be evaluated for metal status, cough, gag, and resolution of the initial problem leading to intubation.

Evaluating for Auto-PEEP in Intubated Patients

Auto-PEEP is an inadvertent level of PEEP that can be caused by insufficient exhalation time, either from inappropriate ventilator settings or restriction to expiratory flow. Auto-PEEP can be detected using the ventilator waveform graphics. When the volume waveform fails to return to baseline following exhalation and before the initiation of the next breath, air is being trapped in the lungs, causing an increase in PEEP. Auto-PEEP can also be evaluated on ventilators where the measured PEEP value is displayed. If the measured PEEP value is higher than the set value, the patient has an increase in auto-PEEP. Auto-PEEP may also make it more difficult for the patient to trigger the ventilator for a breath, causing fatigue and eventual further respiratory failure. For the highly experienced provider, the presence of auto-PEEP can also be detected by auscultation, as the expiratory flow does not cease before the next breath begins.

Evaluating and Interpreting Plateau Pressures in Intubated Patients

Plateau pressure is a measurement that reflects a patient's lung compliance. Plateau pressures are obtained in an intubated patient when all airflow is stopped (at the end of inspiration, but before exhalation). At the end of inspiration, the respiratory therapist can perform an inspiratory hold and the ventilator will calculate the pressure and display a reading for the plateau pressure. Alternatively, the ventilator graphic can be used to measure the pressure at the end of inspiration. The most common reasons for decreased compliance in intubated patients are pneumothorax, pulmonary edema, acute respiratory distress syndrome (ARDS), and pneumonia. Rising plateau pressures indicate worsening lung disease, and when at all possible, changes to ventilator pressures or volumes should be made to keep the plateau from reaching dangerous levels.

Apnea Test Results

An apnea test is a mandatory evaluation for patients with presumed brain death that helps to confirm the absence of brain stem activity. During the test, if no respiration occurs at a $PaCO_2$ of 60 mm Hg (or 20 mm Hg from the patient's baseline), then the patient is considered apneic and the procedure confirms brain death. When evaluating the results of an apnea test in the patient's record, it is important to note the point at which respiration occurs (if any) and the steps taken in the apnea testing procedure. Members of the healthcare team who performed the procedure will log a complete sequence of events for the test procedure as well as the final test findings.

MIP and MEP Results

Prior to initiating extubation, the clinician must first check the patient's record for the MIP and MEP testing results. The patient's record will contain a full explanation of the procedures including equipment used, patient effort and comfort, any adverse events that occurred and the steps taken to correct them, and the final findings. A normal NIF or MIP value is -20mm Hg in a 20 second test, although a MEP value of greater than 40 mm Hg indicates that the patient may be successfully extubated and has enough expiratory respiratory muscle strength to take on the full work of breathing. A normal MEP value also indicates that the patient is likely to have an adequate cough and will be able to successfully clear airway secretions on their own.

Recommend Diagnostic Procedures

Indications and Contraindications for Performing a Thoracentesis

Thoracentesis involves extracting a sample of the pleural fluid via needle aspiration. Thoracentesis is used primarily in the diagnostic process to rule out infections or malignancies. It can also be used as a therapeutic procedure to drain excess pleural fluid prior to placing a chest tube to ease a person's increased work of breathing. The main contraindication to performing a thoracentesis is bleeding. This is especially important if the patient is on anticoagulation therapy, as the bleeding risk is significantly increased. When possible, all anticoagulants should be stopped prior to the procedure and resumed once the procedure is completed. However, this is not an absolute contraindication, and thoracentesis can be completed with extra caution when needed. Infection can occur if the site is not cleaned properly or if it is completed in a non-sterile fashion. Pneumothorax can occur if the lung is punctured during the procedure. Finally, if the needle is incorrectly inserted, it can damage the nerve.

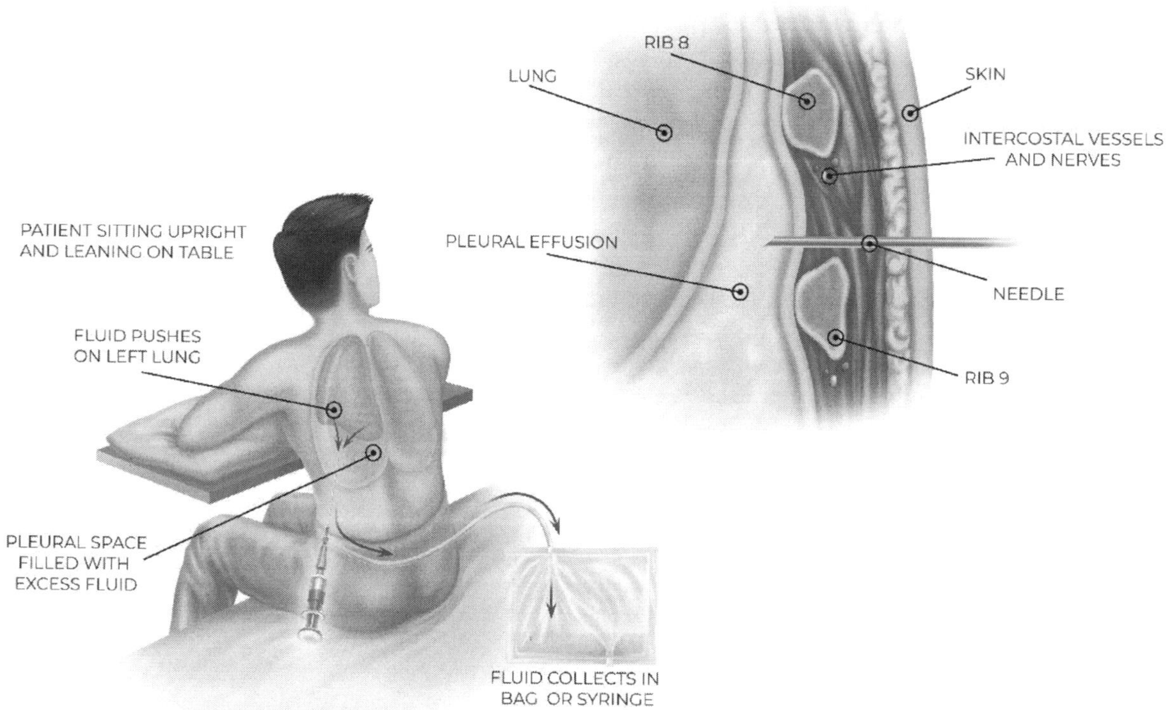

Clinical Signs Indicating the Need for a Sleep Study Recommendation

When a patient presents with key signs and symptoms, these should alert the healthcare professional of a possible sleep disorder. A physical exam of the patient will usually reveal an obese body type (BMI of greater than 40), though someone who is not obese should not immediately be discounted. Men, especially those over the age of 40, have a greater tendency toward obstructive sleep apnea than women do. The patient will usually have a history of snoring on a nightly basis and will usually complain of morning headaches, daytime napping, and fatigue throughout the day. A patient with obstructive sleep apnea will describe being unable to lie flat while sleeping, or sleeping better when propped up by pillows or in a chair. Patients with undiagnosed, severe sleep apnea may even present with pulmonary hypertension or right heart failure from chronic hypoxia.

Recommending a Single-Breath Carbon Monoxide Diffusing Capacity

In its simplest terms, the carbon monoxide diffusing test measures the transfer of gas from the alveoli in the lungs into the blood. Carbon monoxide diffusing capacity represents the diffusing capacity of oxygen across the alveolar-capillary membrane and into the red blood cells. DLCO can be used to help diagnose a number of airway diseases when used in conjunction with other pulmonary function tests. For obstructive diseases, emphysema will be most impacted by a DLCO study. In a patient with emphysema, DLCO will be decreased as the alveolar sacs become overdistended and destroyed. Interstitial lung disease is a restrictive disease that can be identified early with a DLCO study when low lung volumes are also present. If a patient presents with a low DLCO but normal lung volumes, it may indicate pulmonary vascular disease, such as a pulmonary embolism, vasculitis, or pulmonary hypertension.

Closely Monitoring Pulse Oximetry Results in Preterm Infants

Infants who are born premature are at a higher risk of developing complications due to treatment by respiratory therapists. Under normal conditions, the fetus lives in a hypoxic environment in the womb with a PO_2 of approximately 30 mm Hg. When an infant is born premature and is exposed to higher concentrations of oxygen, there is an increase in the PO_2. This increase is even more pronounced as healthcare providers deliver supplemental oxygen in order raise the infant's oxygen levels to what would be considered "normal" for a newborn baby. Even when low concentrations of oxygen are used (21–30%), it is easy to increase PO_2 to levels that are much higher than the fetus maintains in utero. High oxygen levels can be toxic to a premature infant and should be monitored closely, using pulse oximetry. The greatest concern regarding oxygen levels and prematurity is that high or frequently fluctuating oxygen levels can damage the vasculature in the eyes, causing retinopathy of prematurity (ROP). If left untreated, it can cause permanent blindness. High oxygen content can also damage the still developing lung tissue, leading to bronchopulmonary dysplasia and chronic lung disease.

Situations in Which Capnography Should Be Recommended

Capnography can be an invaluable tool for a bedside clinician. It is an excellent trending tool, when used appropriately, to evaluate a patient's condition. It is important to remember that capnography relies on two conditions: ventilation and perfusion. Without both of these components, capnography measurements will be inaccurate. However, when used continuously, capnography can be used to assess a patient perfusion during cardiac arrest. If capnography numbers are present, albeit low, this indicates that compressions are effective enough to produce perfusion through the lungs. During CPR, if there is an abrupt increase in capnography reading, this may indicate that the patient has had return of spontaneous circulation (ROSC). Capnography is routinely used in patients with advanced airways to ensure patency and provide trending of carbon dioxide levels as an alternative to frequent blood draws. Capnography can also be used during conscious sedation to assess whether the patient is overly sedated to the point that respiratory function is impaired.

Indwelling Arterial Line

An indwelling arterial line allows access to the artery for frequent lab draws for arterial blood gases, as well as for continuous monitoring of a patient's systemic blood pressure. Indwelling arterial lines are most frequently placed in the intensive care setting, but can also be placed in the operating room or emergency department. Arterial line placement should be considered for any patient on respiratory support who requires frequent arterial blood gases to monitor respiratory status. Although any indwelling catheter presents an infection risk to the patient, frequent and repeated arterial punctures are not recommended due to risk of bleeding, infection, and arterial laceration. Patients who also require vasoactive pressure support (i.e. dopamine, epinephrine) should have an arterial line placed for continuous blood pressure monitoring and medication titration.

Exhaled NO Testing in the Pulmonary Function Lab

Exhaled nitric oxide testing is part of a complete pulmonary function test that can help determine the degree of inflammation within the pulmonary system. It is also used to measure the degree of baseline severity of chronic inflammation of the airways in asthmatic patients. As swelling and inflammation within the lungs increase, the level of exhaled nitric oxide will also increase. This test can be especially useful to determine whether a patient's asthma is being well controlled with current medication therapy, regardless of symptoms. Uncontrolled inflammation in the lungs can lead to long-term consequences and decreased quality of life for the patient. Monitoring of exhaled nitric oxide is a simple and painless test that gives the provider a great deal of information for managing the patient long term.

Implementing Transcutaneous Monitoring

Transcutaneous monitoring is the process of measuring and trending PCO_2 and PO_2 via skin monitoring probes. It is primarily used in infants and small children, but is becoming more popular in the adult population. Transcutaneous monitoring devices use heat to stimulate blood flow and vasodilation to the area. With the increased blood flow, PCO_2 and PO_2 can be measured. It is commonly used for patients in which minimal stimulation is ideal during mechanical ventilation (neonates and severely ill children), as well as patients requiring frequent monitoring of ventilatory status. It is important to correlate transcutaneous values with an arterial blood gas, as the transcutaneous values are not as precise as those obtained from a blood gas. In neonates and children, transcutaneous monitor probes are often placed on the chest, while in adults probes are placed over areas with thinner tissue layers, such as earlobes.

Benefits and Risks of Invasive Hemodynamic Monitoring

Invasive hemodynamic monitoring can be performed in various ways. An invasive arterial line is a peripherally inserted line (usually the radial or femoral artery) that is used for continuous monitoring of a patient's blood pressure. A pulmonary artery catheter is a centrally inserted line that can be used to measure central venous pressure, pulmonary artery pressure, and pulmonary artery wedge pressure. It allows for continuous monitoring of a patient's fluid status and cardiac output. Either of these lines have the benefit of continuous monitoring for patients with a tenuous hemodynamic status (sepsis, post-op cardiac surgery, etc.) However, any invasive line presents with the risk of infection, as well as bleeding and hemorrhage. With a pulmonary artery catheter, there is also risk of artery perforation, embolism, and blood flow obstruction.

Scenario

A patient with suspected active tuberculosis has been unable to give sufficient sputum samples for testing. What procedures should be recommended?

> To treat tuberculosis, proper diagnosis is critical, along with ensuring proper isolation once the patient is discharged. If the patient is unable to produce sufficient sputum for testing (usually three separate samples are required, 8–12 hours apart), the patient can be given hypertonic saline (either 3% or 7%) to assist in secretion removal. If nebulizers fail to produce a sputum sample, the respiratory therapist can attempt to suction the patient via the nasopharyngeal route to obtain a specimen. If all other options fail, the patient will need to undergo a diagnostic bronchoscopy. The patient will be sedated for the procedure and a physician will insert the

bronchoscope into the lower airways. Saline instillation and airway irrigation can be performed to obtain the needed sample for testing.

Indications for Recommending Static Lung Volumes When Performing a Pulmonary Function Test

Static lung volumes are obtained during a pulmonary function to measure the amount of air in the lungs during specific phases of breathing, as opposed to dynamic volumes that are obtained during inspiration or expiration. Static lung volumes include measurements such as total lung volume (TLV) and residual or reserve volume (RV). Static lung volumes are completed to determine whether a patient has obstructive or restrictive lung disease, as well as severity of the lung disease. Patients with obstructive lung diseases will have difficulty exhaling the full volume of air, making the TLV and RV much higher than expected. Restrictive disease patients will routinely have lower lung volumes, because the higher airway resistance reduces their ability to draw in a deep breath.

Signs and Symptoms That Would Indicate a Sweat Chloride Test

Sweat chloride tests are used to diagnose cystic fibrosis (CF). In cystic fibrosis patients, the amount of chloride in the collected sweat is higher than normal. Cystic fibrosis is often suspected in newborns who present with a meconium ileus (bowel obstruction from thicker than normal meconium). For older children and adults, CF is suspected when there are frequent respiratory infections, coughing or wheezing, greasy or foul-smelling stools, or the diagnosis of infertility in men. Additionally, a salty taste may be evident on the skin when kissed. The test is quick and painless, as a sensor that heats the skin is applied with a device to obtain any sweat that is produced. The test is performed on two different occasions and typically takes less than 30 minutes to complete. Sodium chloride results greater than 60 mmol/L are usually indicative of cystic fibrosis.

Obtaining a Sputum Gram Stain

A sputum gram stain is used to detect and identify bacteria strains in a sputum sample. Sputum gram stains are most commonly used when a pneumonia is suspected, to identify the exact pathogen and ensure that antibiotic coverage is appropriate. Patients who present with a persistent cough; thick or tenacious secretions; foul-smelling secretions; or yellow, green, or brown secretions should be referred for a sputum collection and gram stain. In addition, patients who present with respiratory distress or signs of infection may also need a gram stain. Sputum gram stains can be performed in a clinic or doctor's office and only require the patient to cough up a sample into a sterile container. If there is difficulty coughing secretions out, then a nebulizer with hypertonic saline can be administered to assist with thinning secretions.

Clinical Indications for Recommending an Arterial Blood Gas

Indications for an arterial blood gas include assessing respiratory or metabolic causes of diseases. In the acute care and hospital setting, arterial blood gases should be performed on all patients who require mechanical ventilation, either invasive or noninvasive, or those with suspected impending respiratory failure. Patients presenting with sepsis, liver or renal failure, diabetic ketoacidosis, or other causes of metabolic acidosis should also be ordered for arterial blood gases to assess the level of acid-base dysfunction. In the outpatient setting, arterial blood gases are occasionally taken during sleep studies if a precise level of $PaCO_2$ or PaO_2 is needed to correlate with noninvasive monitoring. In addition, arterial blood gases are often performed on patients with chronic lung disease to assess the level of chronicity, either in the pulmonary function lab as part of a pulmonary function test or prior to high-risk surgery, such as cardiac surgical procedures.

Exhaled CO Monitoring When Recommending a Diffusing Capacity Test

A diffusion capacity test, as part of a pulmonary function test, is used to measure the ability of gases, both CO_2 and O_2, to diffuse or transfer between the alveoli and the blood. In order to be able to diffuse correctly, the alveolar-capillary membrane must remain healthy. This membrane can be altered in certain lung diseases. In most cases, decreased diffusion is caused by either the membrane becoming too thick (such as in pulmonary fibrosis) or the surface area available for diffusion decreasing (such as in emphysema or COPD). In this test, the patient will breathe in a small amount of carbon monoxide. The amount of carbon monoxide that is exhaled is measured and the difference between the two is analyzed. This shows how much of the inhaled gas diffused across the membrane and how much was not able to diffuse and was exhaled instead.

Diagnosing and Evaluating Lung Pleura

Visceral pleura is the layer of tissue that surrounds the lung, while parietal pleura is the layer of tissue that lines the chest wall. Between these two pleural tissue layers is the pleural space. When pleural disease is suspected, including pleural effusion or inflammation, the initial evaluation usually involves a chest x-ray. In many cases, patients may be ordered for a frontal view, as well as a decubitus, x-ray. When the patient lies on his side with the suspected pleural effusion in the dependent position, any fluid will accumulate in this area, making the air-fluid line more prominent. For cases in which additional views or evaluation of pleural diseases need to be recommended, a chest CT can be ordered. The small slices of the lung that can be seen on the chest CT highlights details and locations of pleural disease.

Tests for Patients Admitted to the Hospital with Suspected Pneumonia

When a patient is admitted and suspected of having pneumonia, the initial workup will usually include both a chest x-ray and a complete blood count. The x-ray will determine if any areas of the lung show consolidation consistent with a lobar pneumonia. When an infection is present, the patient will likely have an increase in white blood cell count as the body attempts to fight the infection. If the patient is in moderate to severe respiratory distress, an arterial blood gas with lactate level is beneficial to determine how he is compensating for the decrease in lung function and whether the tissues are receiving enough oxygen. A sputum sample can also be obtained for a sputum gram stain and culture to test for bacteria in the lungs.

Reasons or Conditions for Performing a Bronchoscopy

A bronchoscopy is the insertion of a scope into the airways to perform a visual inspection of the lung tissue and bronchi. Bronchoscopies are usually performed for therapeutic or diagnostic reasons. Therapeutic bronchoscopies are the most common type performed at the hospital bedside. This may be due to thick mucus or atelectasis on chest x-ray. The goal is to identify areas of the lungs that need deep suctioning or irrigation. Samples of fluid may also be obtained to test for bacteria. Diagnostic bronchoscopies are most often performed to identify the reason for a patient's decline in lung function, to obtain a tissue sample for analyses, to diagnose or stage lung cancer, or for routine post lung transplant surveillance. Bronchoscopy is also used to assist in the placement of advanced or surgical airways, especially for verifying placement of tracheostomy tubes.

Performing Pre- and Post-Ductal Saturations in All Newborns

In the first 48–72 hours after birth, major changes in circulation happen in the newborn's body during the transition from intrauterine to extrauterine life. As fetal shunts functionally close, including the ductus arteriosus, oxygen saturations measured pre-ductal and post-ductal should be the same. Prior to discharge, a pre- and post-ductal oxygen saturation test can be performed to ensure that the newborn has transitioned well to the extrauterine environment. If a pre- and post-ductal saturation is performed and there is a difference of greater than 5%, it can be indicative of a shunt remaining open, or, more seriously, a congenital heart defect. Newborns who test positive for a difference of greater than 5% on two tests 8–12 hours apart should be referred for further evaluation and possible echocardiogram.

Diagnostic Procedures for Patients with a Suspected Pulmonary Embolism

If a patient presents with a suspected pulmonary embolism, the initial test is usually a blood test, known as a D-dimer test, to check for levels of protein fragments caused by fibrinolysis of a blood clot. When elevated, it can indicate a clot somewhere in the body but is not exclusively indicative of a pulmonary embolism. If the D-dimer test comes back elevated, or "positive," the patient will have further imaging to test for a blood clot in the lungs. If the use of contrast or radiation is not of immediate concern or is contraindicated, the patient will usually be referred for a spiral CT. This is a quick test with high reliability for diagnosing a pulmonary embolism. If contrast is contraindicated, a perfusion/ventilation scan can be completed. Perfusion/ventilation scans are not as precise, but require less radiation exposure.

Using Ultrasound to Assist with Cardiovascular or Respiratory System Emergencies

The use of ultrasound is rapidly expanding, especially in the emergency departments, intensive care units, and inpatient settings. Ultrasounds are quick and painless and assist with immediate diagnosis of cardiopulmonary emergencies. Effusions, both pulmonary and cardiac, can be determined with ultrasound when used by a trained provider. This diagnosis can lead to quick interventions when needed, including pericardial or pleural drainage via needle or chest tube. When A-lines and B-lines are seen on lung ultrasound, it can help determine or rule out conditions such as COPD, pulmonary embolism, pneumothorax, pleural effusion, and heart failure. Pneumonia can also be identified, especially when unilateral. Ultrasound can also be used to guide providers in the placement of arterial lines and central lines in emergency situations requiring prompt intervention. Ultrasound can be used over the abdomen to assess for massive acute blood loss, such as traumatic liver lacerations or ruptured aorta.

Thermal Ablation

Thermal ablation of the lungs, otherwise known as bronchial thermoplasty, is used to control asthma that has been refractory to other treatments. It is estimated that approximately 5–10% of adults with asthma are considered difficult to treat despite using standard medication therapies. For these patients, treatment involves multiple medications that can have severe side effects with little relief of symptoms. Even with these treatments, the underlying structural changes that occur within the airway smooth muscle are not being addressed. Bronchial thermoplasty is a way to directly minimize the smooth muscle that is in the airway. This minimization limits the ability of these airways to constrict and spasm, a main factor in asthma exacerbations. Thermal ablation should not be considered unless other options have failed and should only be performed by an experienced, trained provider.

Cardiac Biomarkers

The term cardiac biomarkers refers to the hormones, proteins, and enzymes in the blood that are directly affected by cardiac stress, disease, or injury. Cardiac biomarkers include creatinine kinase, myoglobin, creatine kinase-myocardial band (CK-MB), and cardiac troponin. Creatine kinase is an enzyme that, if found in elevated levels, can indicate that a myocardial infarction is underway or has taken place. However, elevated levels can also indicate other diseases and disorders such as musculoskeletal disorders, so it is rarely used independently as a measurement of cardiac health. Similarly, cardiac troponin is a protein that also indicates a myocardial infarction if its level in the blood is significantly elevated. This protein is measurable up to several days after a myocardial infarction, making it the most accurate and widely used cardiac biomarker. Myoglobin is a protein associated with oxygen uptake, which is often measured in conjunction with cardiac troponin to diagnose a myocardial infarction. Lastly, CK-MB is a test measuring two subtypes of phosphocreatine kinase. This test can help diagnose cardiac disorders such as myocardial infarction, ventricular septal defects, and other congenital heart defects of the newborn.

Troubleshooting and Quality Control of Devices, and Infection Control

Assemble and Troubleshoot Devices

Effect of Excess Air in the Syringe on Blood Gas Results

Arterial blood gases are primarily performed to evaluate the oxygenation and ventilation status of a patient. Because of the impact that arterial blood gas results have on a patient's plan of care, it is imperative to obtain accurate results. When obtaining the sample, it is important to immediately remove any air bubbles in the syringe to avoid altering the results. Although in most cases the $PaCO_2$ and pH are only minimally affected, PaO_2 can be greatly affected. Whether it is increased or decreased depends on the original PaO_2 of the blood when drawn from the patient. The PO_2 in the air bubble and the PO_2 in the blood sample exchange via diffusion from high concentration to low concentration. If the patient's blood has a high PO_2, it will appear lower if an air bubble is present, making it seem as if the patient is less oxygenated than he actually is. If the patient has a low PO_2, then the analysis will show a higher value, making the patient seem more oxygenated than he actually is.

Proper Use of an MDI with a Valved Holding Chamber

It is recommended that all patients who take medication via an MDI use a valved holding chamber, also known as a spacer. The MDI should be shaken just prior to administration to ensure proper mixture of medication and propellant. The mouthpiece of the MDI should be inserted into the end of the holding chamber. The patient should be instructed to exhale fully, place the mouthpiece of the holding chamber firmly between the lips, and actuate the MDI. Once actuated, the patient should breathe slowly and deeply through the mouth to fully inhale the medication. At the end of inspiration, an inspiratory hold is performed for 5–10 seconds to improve medication deposition prior to exhalation. The patient should be educated that the use of a holding chamber allows the medication to remain in the chamber so that he can slowly inhale. Without the use of a chamber, the medication is dispersed quickly, and most will deposit on the tongue and in the back of the throat.

Possible Issues Causing a Nitric Oxide Machine to Alarm

Close monitoring is required for patients receiving inhaled nitric oxide therapy. The half-life of nitric oxide, once inhaled, is only about 6 seconds, so alarms of potential administration disruption should be investigated immediately. One of the most common alarms that presents during administration is when the NO and NO_2 monitors fail to display a number. When this alarm activates, it means that the machine is unable to calculate the values that are being sampled from the patient's breathing circuit. Although not common, the sample line, filter, and water trap should be assessed to ensure that they have not become disconnected from the device or the patient circuit. The most common cause is condensation buildup, either in the water trap, the filter, or within the sample line itself. If this occurs, the water trap should be emptied and the filter and sample line should be replaced. To prevent this alarm, the water trap should be emptied routinely and the sample line should be disconnected or a sample line filter placed whenever a nebulized treatment is administered.

Scenario

A patient is on a ventilator in SIMV-PRVC. The high-pressure alarm is active. Describe possible causes of the alarm.

When using PRVC, the provider sets a tidal volume to be delivered, and the ventilator adjusts the pressure required to reach this volume. The provider will also set a high-pressure limit. If the high-pressure limit is reached, the full set total volume will not be delivered, which can adversely impact the patient's ventilatory status. For this reason, it is critical to determine the cause of the high-pressure alarm. The respiratory therapist should investigate the patient's status. If a patient is anxious, biting the endotracheal tube, or breath holding and actively fighting the ventilator breaths, he needs to be calmed, either by redirection or medication. The high-pressure alarm can also be triggered by kinking or bending the ventilator tubing or endotracheal tube, or by secretions in the tube that need to be suctioned out. The high-pressure alarm can also be activated by changes in the patient's lung compliance, such as bronchospasm, atelectasis, or pulmonary edema.

Causes of Temperature Fluctuations in a Heated, Humidified System

Many respiratory devices are heated and humidified by a heating device since the upper airway is either bypassed (as in endotracheal tubes and tracheostomy tubes) or the flow is too great for the upper airway to properly humidify and heat (high-flow nasal cannula and CPAP/BiPAP). Many hospital-grade heated humidifiers operate on a feedback loop; the system monitors the airway temperature just prior to the patient interface and heats or cools the water chamber depending on this temperature. Disruptions in these monitoring temp probes can cause temperature fluctuations. First, the temperature probes should be assessed for proper placement within the circuit. There also needs to be air flowing through the circuit so that it flows over the temperature probes. Outside sources of heat or cooling (such as incubators or fans) can change the temperature of the air at the temperature probe, causing major temperature fluctuations. Condensation on the temperature probes can also cause false readings and temperature swings.

Contraindications for Heat and Moisture Exchangers (HME)

Providing humidification to the respiratory system is important to maintain homeostasis. However, additional evaluations are necessary to ensure that the use of an HME is safe. If the patient has thick or copious secretions, there is an increased risk of obstructing the filter, and therefore the airway as well. In addition, the manufacturer suggestions should be read to ensure that the minimum exhaled tidal volume is being met. If the exhaled tidal volume is below the manufacturer recommendation, the patient will not get the required humidification. It is also important that the patient not be hypothermic, as he will not exhale the proper heat that the HME must maintain to function properly. An HME is also inappropriate for patients receiving continuous nebulization or other forms of humidification. Finally, an HME needs to be removed prior to administering an intermittent nebulizer.

Preanalytical Causes of Blood Gas Errors

Preanalytical errors are defined as errors that occur before the blood is analyzed. This usually includes errors that occur during the sampling or transport process. The most common preanalytical error occurs when air bubbles are not properly removed from the syringe. If the top layer of blood is "frothy" or if there are air bubbles visible in the syringe after drawing the sample, they should be removed immediately. During the drawing process, it is also possible that venous blood is drawn instead of arterial. When blood is filling the syringe, it should be pulsatile and able to fill the syringe on its own. If the blood is unable to fill the syringe without applying pressure, a venous sample should be suspected. The sample should be analyzed as soon as possible to prevent changes due to continued metabolism. Finally, when using a heparinized syringe, any visible heparin, whether liquid or powder, should be removed or completely mixed into the sample.

Components to Check When Troubleshooting an Oxygen Analyzer

Oxygen analyzers (independent from those inside devices such as ventilators or BiPAP machines) help the respiratory therapist determine the precise oxygen percentage being delivered to the patient. Prior to using an oxygen analyzer, it should first be calibrated to ensure that it will read the correct FiO_2. Different analyzers may differ slightly in the process, but in general, the process will include analyzing at 21% oxygen (room air sample) and then at 100% oxygen. If either of these numbers read differently, they should be adjusted on the analyzer to match the FiO_2 percentage being analyzed. After analyzing, if there are still issues with the analyzer, the individual replaceable parts should be checked and replaced as needed. Depending on the manufacturer, these parts may include: batteries, electrodes, analyzer cord, and membranes.

Problems Causing Measurement Errors When Using a Hemoximeter

Hemoximetry works by placing a device on a finger or earlobe and directing a beam of light through the body part. On the other side of the finger or earlobe is a device that measures the amount of light passing through. From this, it can be determined how much oxygen is being carried in the blood and to the tissues. Measurement errors can cause falsely low or falsely high hemoglobin or oxyhemoglobin levels. Inaccurate elevated hemoglobin readings can be caused by an abnormally high level of fetal hemoglobin (high fetal hemoglobin can be normal in preterm infants) and increased bilirubin levels (which can indicate liver failure in adults). Low readings of hemoglobin or oxyhemoglobin can be seen in those with sickle cell disease, increased blood lipid levels, or incomplete hemolysis of blood.

Considerations When Using a Pulse Oximeter

Pulse oximetry is the standard, noninvasive way to monitor a patient's oxygenation level. Since there are many manufacturers of pulse oximetry equipment, it is important to make sure that the disposable or attachable probes are compatible with the manufacturer of the pulse ox machine or monitor. There are also different pulse ox sizes and shapes, depending on patient size and probe placement location. When initially placing a pulse oximeter probe, allow time for calibration so that the recorded number is accurate. The sensor should also not be too tight as this can restrict blood flow to the area and give a false reading. If the probe is too loose, it may not be able to obtain a proper signal, can fall off of the patient, or may read improperly due to ambient light.

Factors Affecting the Reading of a Pulse Oximeter

There are many factors that can affect the reading of a pulse oximeter and will require an arterial blood gas to correlate. Certain abnormal forms of hemoglobin, such as carboxyhemoglobin and methemoglobin, will read as highly saturated hemoglobin on a pulse oximeter. Although the hemoglobin is highly saturated, these are not saturated with oxygen. In these cases, patients can be very hypoxic at the tissue level with saturations of 100%. Ambient light, especially fluorescent light, can interfere with the wavelengths of light and provide false readings. Dark nail polish can prevent light from crossing the nail bed, providing an inaccurately low reading, as can darkly pigmented skin. Poor perfusion to the probe site will hinder the probe's ability to read properly, providing an inaccurate reading and various SpO_2 recordings. Anemic patients with low hematocrit or patients who have recently received intravascular dyes can also give off false low readings.

Causes of Ventilator Asynchrony

Causes of patient-ventilator asynchrony can be divided into three types: flow, trigger, or cycle asynchrony. Flow asynchrony is usually caused when the patient's flow demand is higher than the flow being delivered by the ventilator. This reduced flow will make the patient feel air hunger and attempt to pull more air. Trigger asynchrony can present in multiple ways, some of which include double triggering, missed triggering, auto triggering, or delayed triggering. In any event, trigger asynchrony is when the start of the ventilator breath and the start of the patient breath do not correlate. Cycle asynchrony occurs when inspiration is terminated by the ventilator either before or after the patient is ready to exhale. This type of asynchrony is usually caused by an inappropriately set inspiratory time, either too long or too short.

Interventions Assisting in Minimizing Auto-PEEP

Auto-PEEP is a result of incomplete exhalation, and can be caused intrinsically by the patient's pulmonary disease or extrinsically as a result of mechanical ventilation settings. To combat intrinsic causes of auto-PEEP, bronchopulmonary hygiene can reduce the buildup of secretions that can prevent airflow. Bronchodilators can be administered if bronchoconstriction is the primary cause, such as in asthma. From a ventilator management perspective, a decrease in inspiratory time, set rate, or tidal volume can all increase the expiratory time, allowing for greater exhalation and decreasing auto-PEEP. Increasing the set inspiratory flow or exhalation time can also provide increased ventilation. Another method is increasing the set PEEP to equal the auto-PEEP, which can help stent the lower airways open. Assessment of equipment should also be done to ensure the correct size endotracheal tube and ventilator circuit are being used to accommodate for larger volumes of gas exchange.

Causes of Ventilator Auto-Triggering

The term auto-triggering refers to the ventilator initiating quick, frequent breaths. It occurs when the ventilator senses what appears to be patient initiation but is not. In some cases the sensitivity on the ventilator is set to sensitive and it perceives any movement of the ventilator circuit as the patient's. Another common cause of auto-triggering is condensation buildup in the circuit. As the water builds in the dependent portion of the circuit, it begins to move back and forth with circuit movements or ventilator breaths, triggering the ventilator to initiate a breath. Draining this water will easily solve this issue. Other possible causes of auto-triggering include small leaks or holes in the circuit, unsecured tubing connections, and even a hyperdynamic patient whose heart is contracting so forcefully that it can be picked up by the ventilator.

Cycle Asynchrony

Cycle asynchrony is caused when the set inspiratory time on the ventilator differs from the patient's desired inspiratory time. It occurs most commonly during pressure ventilation. Cycle asynchrony is most easily diagnosed by assessing the waveform graphics. If the inspiratory time on the ventilator is set too short, a notch will be observed after the end of the set inspiratory time, indicating the patient's desire to keep inspiring (double triggering). If the inspiratory time is set too long, a notch will be visible on the graphic prior to the end of inspiration. This indicates the patient's desire to exhale while the ventilator is still delivering a breath. In order to correct cycle asynchrony, adjust the set inspiratory time or the cycle percentage time to better meet the patient's demands.

Initial Ventilator Set-Up

Prior to initiation of mechanical ventilation, the healthcare team should determine the correct method and settings for the patient. First, it should be determined whether the patient can be sustained on noninvasive ventilation or if intubation is required. If intubation is required, the type and size of the endotracheal tube should be determined, along with risk factors for intubation, such as previous airway surgeries, obesity, or other factors that could make intubation difficult. The choice of ventilator mode and level of needed support should be decided, along with specific ventilator settings, such as targeted tidal volume based on ideal body weight and initial set respiratory rate, inspiratory time, FiO_2 and PEEP. Prior to leaving the patient, it is also important to check that all alarms are adjusted and set to detect changes in the patient's respiratory pattern or compliance.

Aspects Influencing Ventilator Response Time

Ventilator response time is mostly influenced by the set trigger sensitivity. When deciding on trigger sensitivity, set the most sensitive trigger that does not allow for auto triggering. If the sensitivity is set to difficult, the patient will have to work harder to trigger a breath. Other factors that can affect the ventilator response time to the patient's desire for a breath include air trapping, which can make it difficult for the patient to generate the flow change needed to trigger the ventilator. Additional dead space within the circuit, including tubing that is too long and additional items added to the circuit, such as end tidal devices, MDI adaptors, and nebulizers mean that the patient must overcome this additional volume to trigger the ventilator for a breath. Malfunctions can also occur if there is an issue with the valve not opening to allow for breathing, but this is rare with appropriate set-up and maintenance.

Types of Interface Devices That Can Be Used with Noninvasive Ventilation Set-Ups

The most common patient interfaces for use with noninvasive ventilation are the nasal masks and the oronasal mask. For a patient presenting in acute respiratory failure, the oronasal mask is the best option if the patient is able to tolerate it. The mask completely covers the mouth and nose to ensure complete airway coverage and provide the best pressure delivery. The next best option is the nasal mask, but it can be difficult to deliver the appropriate pressures if the patient opens his mouth or is a primary mouth breather. For home use, the most common interfaces in addition to those listed above are nasal pillows. Nasal pillows sit in the nares without covering the external nose. The choice of interface for home or long-term use will depend on the patient's breathing habits (mouth or nose breather) and what the patient finds the most comfortable and will be most likely to stay compliant with. Additional interfaces include the total face mask (covering the entire face from the forehead to the chin) and the helmet (which covers the entire head).

Common Complications Occurring During Noninvasive Pressure Ventilation

The most common complication for noninvasive ventilation is patient discomfort. Although this may appear unimportant, it often leads to the patient being noncompliant with the therapy. Claustrophobia is the main cause of noncompliance and can be relieved with different interfaces. Skin breakdown or pressure sores can develop if the apparatus is applied too tightly or if it used for an extended period of time without a skin barrier applied. Drying of mucus membranes from improperly humidified air can lead to sinus issues and bleeding. Gastric discomfort can occur from air being forced into the stomach. Serious complications can involve aspiration from vomiting while wearing a noninvasive interface, pneumothorax from pressure and lung overdistension, and decreased blood pressure from overdistension of the lungs, resulting in decreased venous return.

Main Pressures/Volumes Assessed and Adjusted When Using Lung Protective Strategies During Ventilation

Mechanical ventilation, although a life-saving intervention for a patient unable to breathe on his own, can have consequences when applied incorrectly. Pressures used during mechanical ventilation can cause damage to lung tissue. In order to prevent damage, respiratory therapists need to observe and track four important pressures. Transpulmonary pressure is the pressure difference between the alveolar pressure and the intrapleural pressure. This pressure is most closely related to plateau pressure measured on mechanical ventilators. Ideally, plateau pressure should be kept at or below 28 cm H_2O. Tidal volumes should be kept between 4 and 8 ml/kg of ideal body weight. When in pressure control ventilation, pressures should be adjusted to keep tidal volumes within this range. PEEP should be kept at an adequate level to prevent lungs from becoming derecruited during exhalation. An optimal PEEP study can be performed to find the ideal PEEP for the patient. Finally, the driving pressure (difference between plateau pressure and PEEP) should be kept below 15 cm H_2O.

Causes of Changes in End Tidal CO_2 Readings

Both ventilation and perfusion are necessary for an accurate CO_2 measurement. Therefore, changes in CO_2 readings can be divided into two main groups: changes in ventilation and changes in perfusion. If the patient's lung compliance or resistance changes dramatically, as in a bronchospasm, pneumothorax, pleural effusion, pulmonary edema, or change in abdominal pressures, CO_2 readings can change quickly. Changes in perfusion will also create sudden changes in CO_2 readings, such as pericardial effusion, pericardial tamponade, pulmonary embolism, or cardiac arrest. If the patient has an advanced airway and there is a sudden change in end tidal CO_2, it is important to assess external factors, such as disconnection from the ventilator tubing, tube occlusion due to kinking or secretions, or an end tidal malfunction such as secretions or water in the sampling line. The normal capnogram is a waveform that represents the varying CO_2 level throughout the breath cycle:

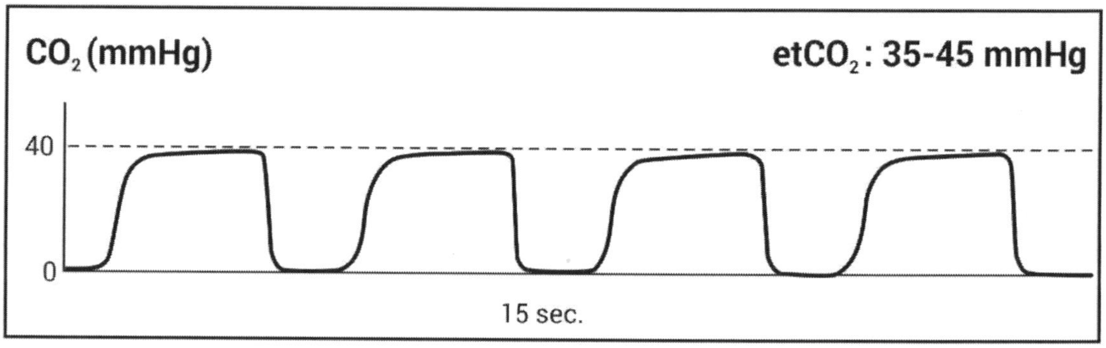

Role of Ventilator Graphics in Troubleshooting Patient-Ventilator Asynchrony

There are four phases of patient ventilator asynchrony that can be identified using ventilator graphics. Trigger asynchrony can be caused by inappropriate trigger sensitivity and can be seen with a double trigger or increase in pressure at the end of inspiration. Flow asynchrony is caused when the set flow is inconsistent with the patient's needs, usually too low for patient demand. Termination asynchrony occurs when the end of inspiration happens earlier or later than the patient needs. Finally, expiratory asynchrony happens when the expiratory phase is too short or too long to meet the expiratory need of the patient. By identifying each of these phases on a ventilator graphic, the respiratory therapist is able to isolate where the asynchrony is occurring and make adjustments to meet the patient's demand.

Placing a Nasal Cannula on an Adult Patient

When placing a nasal cannula on an adult patient, the clinician must first confirm a written order for oxygen therapy as well as confirm the liter flow. When using a nasal cannula without humidity, the clinician will gather the necessary equipment including a nipple or "Christmas tree" adapter and an adult-sized nasal cannula. The clinician will introduce themselves to the patient and explain the procedure. Then the clinician will screw the nipple adapter onto the room's flow meter and attach the end of the nasal cannula. Then, the clinician will insert the nasal cannula into the patient's nares, with the prongs following the curve of the patient's anatomy. The clinician will then tighten the nasal cannula as needed for patient comfort and turn on the flow meter to the predetermined liter flow. If humidity needs to be added, a nipple adapter is not necessary. The clinician will pierce the neck of the humidifier by screwing on the humidifier's flow meter adapter. The humidifier is then screwed onto the flow meter after first removing a nipple adapter if one is present. Save the nipple adapter for future use by securing it at the bedside. Attach the nasal cannula tubing to the humidifier and place the nasal cannula on the patient. Then turn the flow meter onto the desired liter flow.

Extension Tubing with a Nasal Cannula

Patients who require continuous oxygen therapy and/or patients who require oxygen therapy on exertion will likely require extension tubing in order to wear their nasal cannula as they move around their hospital room or home. Extension tubing is used with the use of small adapters that attach between the extension tubing and nasal cannula tubing (or between extension tubing lengths if more than one is required). It is important to note that there is a limit to how many extension tubing lengths can be used. Check your facility's policies and procedures as well as with the guidelines of the manufacturer of the nasal cannula and tubing to ensure that the correct number of extension tubing lengths are used. The use of excessive amounts of extension tubing can result in reduced flow delivered to the patient and subsequent shortness of breath.

Pediatric and Neonatal Patients on Nasal Cannulas

When placing a nasal cannula on a pediatric or neonatal patient, the clinician must first choose an appropriately sized nasal cannula. This may require measurement of the nares with the cannula manufacturer's measuring devices. It is important to measure the patient's nares to ensure a snug fit without flaring or completely occluding the nares. Nasal cannulas often need to be secured to neonatal and pediatric patients. This can be achieved by using facility-approved skin protective adhesive devices such as Tegaderm. Check with your facility's policies and procedures to determine which adhesive substance is appropriate. The clinician will then place the Tegaderm or other adhesive tape to the nasal cannula and patient's cheeks, ensuring that the nasal cannula will not become dislodged. The patient's skin will need to be evaluated regularly for breakdown.

Troubleshooting a Nasal Cannula

Patient Is Experiencing Reduced Flow

When a patient is complaining of reduced flow while using a nasal cannula, the clinician must first check all connections in the circuit and ensure that the flow meter is turned on and functioning. If any disconnections are observed between the nipple adapter and tubing or between the lengths of extension tubing (if present), then the clinician should reattach the disconnection. The clinician should also tighten all other connections to ensure that there is not a leak in the circuit. If the patient is using a humidifier, the clinician should ensure that it is functioning properly. Finally, the clinician should check to make sure that the patient is not using excessive amounts of extension tubing, which can result in reduced flow. If the clinician cannot find a problem with the equipment and the flow is still reduced, then he or she should replace the equipment.

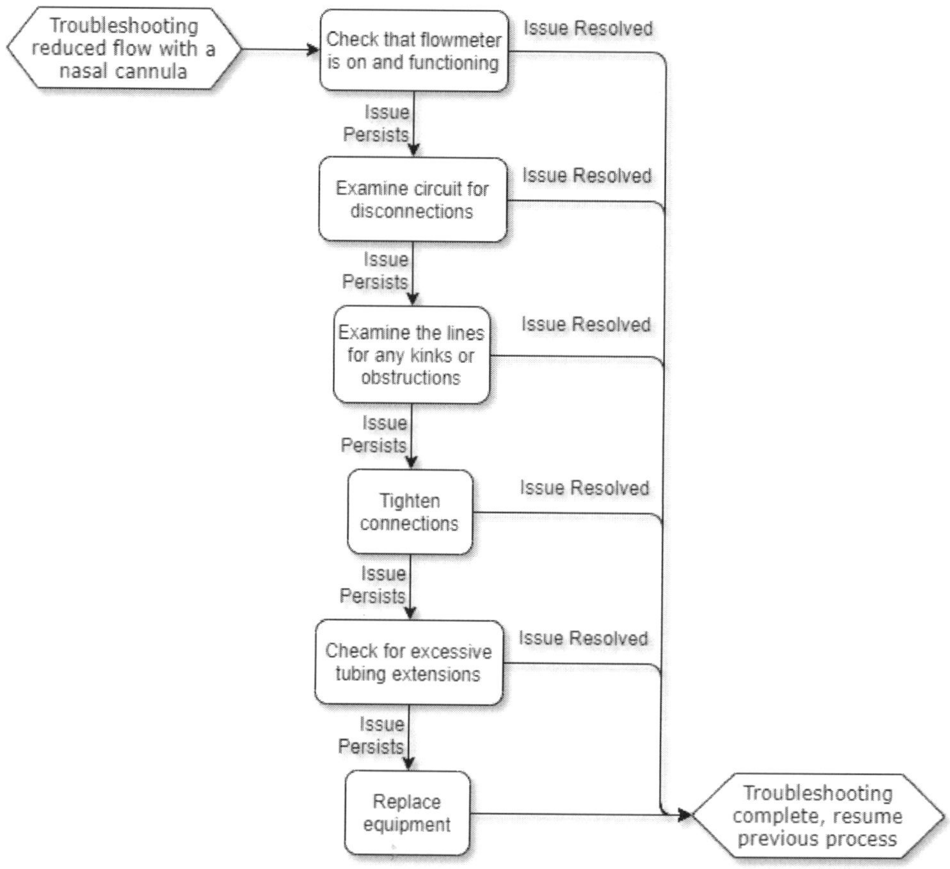

HUMIDIFIER IS MAKING A HIGH-PITCHED SQUEALING NOISE

If a nasal cannula with humidifier is making a high-pitched squealing noise, it is likely that there is a kink in the system. The clinician should first check the entire length of the circuit, correcting all kinks in the tubing. If no kinks are found, the clinician should then visually inspect the circuit for other sources of obstruction such as mucus plugging in the nasal prongs, dirt or debris in the tubing, or tubing that is kinked due to furniture being placed on top of it. If no obstruction is found, the equipment should be replaced.

HUMIDIFIER IS BUBBLING EXCESSIVELY, BECOMING DISTENDED, AND EMITTING A HIGH-PITCHED NOISE

When using a nasal cannula with a humidifier, it is important to ensure that the flow rate is not too high for the humidifier. Refer to your facility's policies and procedures as well as the manufacturer's guidelines for liter flow limitations for your facility-approved humidifier. If a humidifier is starting to become distended, is emitting a high-pitched noise, and is bubbling excessively, the clinician should suspect that the liter flow is too high for the humidifier. When the flow meter is set at an excessive flow rate, usually greater than 8 liters per minute, the humidifier becomes overwhelmed and backflow causes it to distend, make noise, and bubble loudly. The clinician should reduce the flow rate and observe changes in the system. If the problem is solved, then the patient may need to change to a high-flow nasal cannula or other high-flow oxygen system to provide them with the liter flow they require. If reducing the liter flow does not solve the problem, the system should be checked for leaks and kinks. If none are present, the equipment should be replaced.

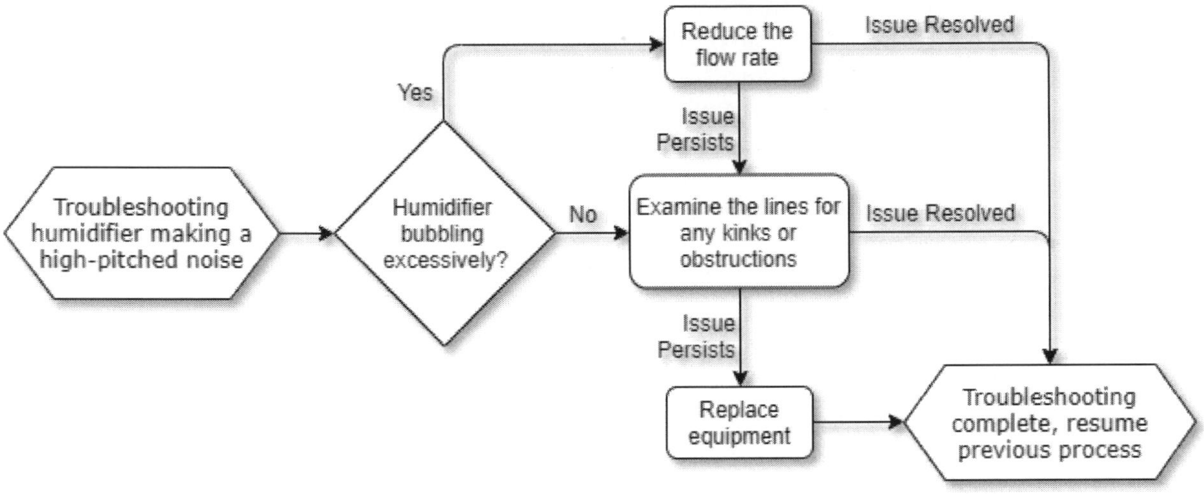

Heated High-Flow Nasal Cannula

When placing a patient on a heated high-flow nasal cannula, the clinician will first need to confirm the physician's order. Next, the clinician will gather the necessary equipment including the heated high-flow nasal cannula, oxygen blender, circuitry, sterile water source, and humidifier. For neonatal and pediatric patients, the clinician will need to measure the patient's nares and choose the corresponding size of nasal cannula. If the nasal cannula prongs are too large, complications such as tissue breakdown and hypoventilation can occur. Setup of a heated high-flow nasal cannula can vary based on your facility's equipment. Refer to your facility's policies and procedures for setting up a heated high-flow nasal cannula. Generally speaking, the clinician will attach the inspiratory circuit to the humidifier and attach a shorter length of circuit from the oxygen blender to the humidifier. The clinician will attach a sterile water bag to the humidifier. Ensure that the humidifier is plugged into a power source and turned on, with the temperature set to the desired level. Connect the heated wires to the corresponding outlets in the circuit. Ensure that the oxygen blender is plugged into an adequate gas source. Dial in the flow rate on the flow meter and adjust the FiO_2 on the oxygen blender. Then place the nasal cannula prongs into the patient's nares, following the curve of the anatomy. Finally, document the procedure.

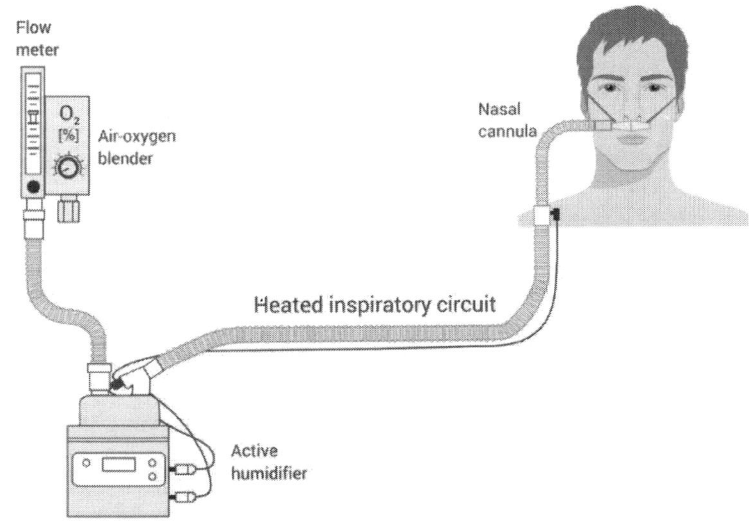

Identifying Candidates for Heated High-Flow Nasal Cannula Therapy

Heated high-flow nasal cannulas can be used in patients of all ages, including adults, children, and neonates. In adult and pediatric populations, heated high-flow nasal cannulas are commonly used for patients who require high oxygen flow rates. Traditional nasal cannulas with or without humidifiers have limits on the flow rates that can be successfully delivered to the patient. Excessive flow rates on traditional nasal cannulas can also lead to drying of the nasopharyngeal mucosa and subsequent patient discomfort. Neonatal patients are often placed on heated high-flow nasal cannulas as an alternative to CPAP because heated high-flow nasal cannulas are associated with fewer instances of skin breakdown and other complications while still delivering positive end expiratory pressure, humidity, and oxygen to the patient.

Self-Inflating Resuscitator

A self-inflating resuscitation bag, also known as an Ambu bag, does not require airflow to inflate. Instead, the bag remains inflated until the bag is squeezed. When using a self-inflating resuscitation bag, the clinician must first ensure that the bag is attached to an oxygen source. Next, the clinician will turn the flow meter up to 15 liters per minute. A self-inflating bag can be used by attaching the adapter to an endotracheal tube or tracheostomy tube, or it can be used with a mask for patients who do not have an artificial airway. When using a mask with the self-inflating resuscitation bag, the clinician must stand at the head of the bed and secure the mask onto the patient's face using E-C hand placement.

E-C Hand Placement

E-C hand placement refers to the position of a clinician's fingers during ventilation and resuscitation with a bag and mask. With this type of ventilation, the clinician's thumb and index finger of one hand form a C shape clamped around the mask on the patient's face. Their hand makes an E shape as their remaining fingers follow the curve of the patient's jaw, lifting it slightly. This hand placement allows for a proper seal, and the E position helps to lift the jaw into the sniffing position. This ensures an open and patent airway. Once the hand position is correct, the clinician squeezes the bag with their other hand and observes the patient for chest rise during ventilation.

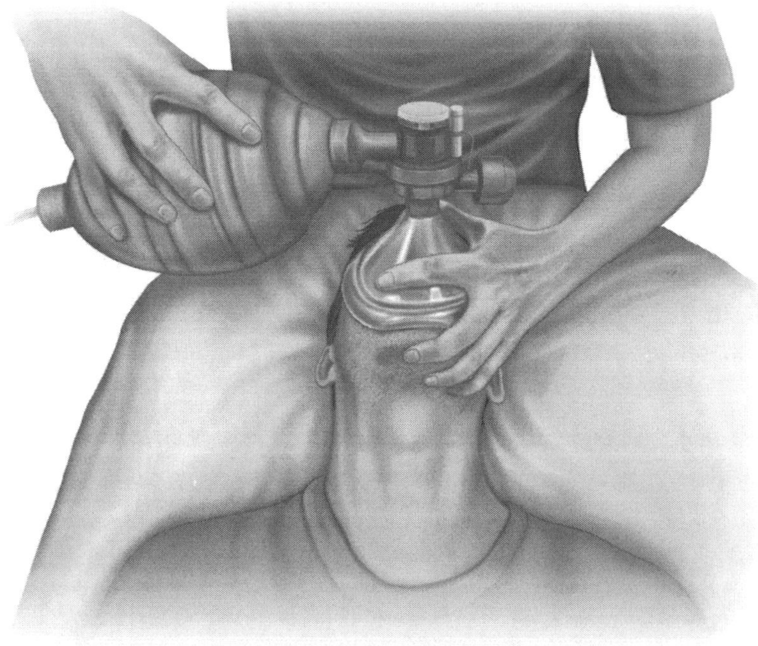

Flow-Inflating Resuscitator

A flow-inflating resuscitation bag requires a gas source for inflation. The bag looks similar to a deflated balloon until it is attached to a gas source and it begins to inflate. Equipment may vary depending on the types used at your facility. Refer to your facility's policies and procedures for proper flow-inflating resuscitation bag setup. Generally speaking, the flow into the bag is adjusted by turning a wheel located on the base of the bag. The delivered pressures are adjusted by decreasing or increasing the strength of squeezing the bag. Monitor the attached pressure manometer to ensure that the patient is being ventilated at adequate but not excessive pressures. Increasing the flow will cause the bag to inflate more, whereas decreasing the flow will cause the bag to begin to deflate. A flow-inflating bag can be used by attaching the adapter to an endotracheal tube or tracheostomy tube, or it can be used with a mask for patients who do not have artificial airways. When using a mask, the clinician must stand at the head of the bed and secure the mask onto the patient's face using E-C hand placement. Then the clinician squeezes the bag with their other hand and observes the patient for chest rise during ventilation as well as watching the pressure manometer.

Troubleshooting a Self-Inflating Resuscitation Bag

No Chest Rise Is Observed

If no chest rise is observed during ventilation with a self-inflating resuscitation bag, the clinician should first check their E-C hand position for correct placement. This hand placement allows for a proper seal and helps to lift the jaw into the sniffing position. If chest rise is still not observed, the clinician should reposition the mask and replace their hands into the E-C position, lifting the jaw gently. Chest rise may be absent if the patient's airway is not fully open or if there is not an adequate seal between the mask and the patient's face.

Delivered Pressures Are Low and the Bag Is Partially Deflated

When ventilating a patient with a flow-inflating resuscitation bag, it is essential that the clinician simultaneously monitor the airflow into the bag and the pressures delivered to the patient as displayed on the attached pressure manometer. If the pressures are low and the bag is partially deflated, the bag is not receiving enough flow from the flow meter or oxygen blender and the patient is not being adequately ventilated. First, attempt to increase the flow by adjusting the flow wheel on the base of the bag. If that doesn't solve the problem, check all connections to ensure a tight fit. If leaks are suspected or if the problem cannot be identified quickly, replace the resuscitation bag.

Delivered Pressures Are High and the Patient Is Difficult to Ventilate

If a clinician needs to squeeze the flow-inflating resuscitation bag with greater force or if the delivered pressures are high, then there may be an obstruction in the system. The clinician should check for obstructions in the tube by suctioning out any mucus plugs or secretions. The clinicians should also check for any kinks or obstructions in the tubing or circuit. If no obstructions are found in the endotracheal tube or the resuscitation equipment, the clinician should then visually inspect the patient, noting any tracheal shift or other abnormalities that could indicate complications such as a pneumothorax. If a complication such as pneumothorax or severe bronchospasm is present, it must be treated immediately in order to continue with successful ventilation and resuscitation.

Troubleshooting Self-Inflating and Flow-Inflating Resuscitation Bags with a Mask and Endotracheal Tube When the Patient Is Becoming Increasingly Difficult to Ventilate

If a clinician needs to squeeze a resuscitation bag with greater force, then there is some form of obstruction in the system. For intubated patients, the clinician should first ensure that the patient is not biting the endotracheal tube, causing an obstruction. If the patient is biting the tube, placement of an oral airway can be helpful. This "bite block" keeps the patient's airway open and patent and prevents the patient from biting down on the tube. The tube can also be suctioned to remove any mucus plugs or secretions clogging the tube. For patients who are not using an endotracheal tube, the clinician should check their hand position and ensure a tight seal on the patient's mask. The clinician should evaluate the patient's airway for patency. If no obstructions are found in the tube or airway, the clinician should then visually inspect the patient, noting any tracheal shift or other abnormalities that could indicate complications such as pneumothorax. If a complication such as pneumothorax or severe bronchospasm is present, it must be treated immediately in order to continue successful ventilation and resuscitation.

Hyperinflation Devices

Some patients are at risk for lung consolidation, such as patients undergoing abdominal or thoracic surgery. These patients benefit from hyperinflation devices such as incentive spirometers. An incentive spirometer is a device in which the patient places the mouthpiece in their mouth, ensures a tight seal with their lips, and then inhales slowly for several seconds, keeping the indicator within the target zone. The process is typically repeated 10 times per hour. This therapy promotes diaphragmatic breathing and prevents atelectasis in the lung bases. After the initial instruction, the patient is often able to perform the task independently throughout their hospital stay. A pillow can be pressed to the stomach if the patient's incisions are painful during therapy.

Testing Equipment in a Pulmonary Function Laboratory

A pulmonary function laboratory contains several pieces of equipment that measures lung volumes and flow. Equipment varies widely between facilities, so the clinician should refer to their facility's policies and procedures for the proper use and maintenance of their equipment. Generally speaking, pulmonary function testing can include equipment such as a body plethysmograph, which can measure lung volumes and flows, diffusion capacity, and nitrogen washout; a simple spirometer, which also measures lung volumes and flows; and exhaled nitric oxide measuring equipment, which indicates the level of inflammation in the patient's lungs. Exhaled nitric oxide measurement is especially helpful in the diagnosis and treatment of inflammatory lung diseases such as asthma.

Ensure Infection Prevention

Types of Isolation

Contact isolation is used to prevent the spread of disease that is only transmitted by direct or indirect contact. It involves standard precautions, plus the use of gloves and isolation gowns whenever providing patient care or when contact with the patient's environment is anticipated. When possible, the patient should also be placed in a private room. Droplet isolation is used to prevent the transmission of diseases, such as the flu virus, that are transmitted in droplet form. The patient should be placed in a private room and a mask should be used whenever providing care for the patient or entering the patient's environment. Airborne precautions require the use of a respirator or N-95 mask. The patient should be isolated in a private, negative-pressure room. Care should be taken to limit transport of the patient through the hospital and unnecessary personnel from entering the patient's room.

Ways That Infections Are Transmitted

Understanding how infections are transmitted is essential to preventing their spread from patient to patient within the hospital. Contact transmission is organism transfer from person to person (direct) or from an infected object to a person (indirect). Droplet transmission involves passing infection to others through sneezing and coughing. Transmission of this infection is usually limited to about three feet. Airborne transmission involves drops of contaminated fluid. Due to the small size of the particles, they can be spread over long distances, so special room filters and negative pressure systems should be used to prevent this spread of infection. Common vehicle transmission is the passing of infection through food or water. Salmonella is a common example of this type of transmission. Finally, vector-borne transmission is the passing of infection from one host to another via a carrier, such as infections that result from insect bites.

Cleaning, Disinfecting, and Sterilizing Equipment

Cleaning equipment is the most basic form of interrupting transmission of infection through devices. Usually, a basic cleaning solvent and water or a specialized cleaning wipe, such as antiseptic or bleach wipes, is used to remove foreign matter from the device. A basic cleaning process is usually the first step prior to disinfecting or sterilizing in order to remove excess debris from equipment. Since soaps are unable to kill most bacteria, a higher level of infection control is usually needed. Disinfecting kills most pathogens and microorganisms when a high-level disinfectant is used. The highest level of infection control is sterilization. During the sterilizing process, all forms of microbes are destroyed. Sterilization is required for many hospital tools, including operating room equipment and anything used invasively at the patient bedside.

Deciding Between Disposable and Reusable Equipment

There are different factors to discuss when considering whether to use disposable or reusable equipment. The issue of infection risk and patient safety is a top priority. If equipment cannot be properly disinfected or sterilized between patients, disposable equipment may be necessary. It is impossible to make certain types of equipment disposable, so the only choice is reusable. It is also important to consider the availability of hospital resources, both equipment and personnel. For sterilization procedures, it may take hours to clean and sterilize equipment. Finally, cost is always an issue in healthcare, and the cost of disposable versus reusable material may sway the decision.

Donning and Doffing PPE

Personal protective equipment (PPE), including gowns, masks, and gloves, is often used when a patient is in an isolation room due to infectious and contagious disease. PPE is also commonly used for situations that are inherently messy such as traumas and bedside procedures. When putting on (donning) PPE, the clinician first undergoes hand hygiene. Then, the clinician dresses in the appropriate PPE. The clinician should not touch their face after donning the equipment. Once the procedure is over, the clinician must carefully discard the equipment in the patient's room. This is achieved by first taking off (doffing) their gown and gloves "inside out" so as to not contaminate their hands with biohazardous material. Then they remove their mask and discard it. Finally, they perform hand hygiene a second time. If a respirator is used instead of a mask, it should be removed and discarded outside of the patient's room.

Perform Quality Control Procedures

Quality Control Measures Related to Blood Gas Analyzers

There are three electrodes in most blood gas analyzers. The Severinghaus electrode is used to analyze PCO_2 measurements, the Clark electrode is used to measure the PO_2, and the Sanz electrode is used in pH analysis. To make sure that these analyzers are working properly, it is important to perform routine calibration tests. The frequency of calibration depends on the manufacturer, but many require calibration at least every 24 hours. To perform a calibration, solutions with known values are run through as a blood gas would be analyzed. It is typical to run at least two solutions, one with low values and one with high values. Performing these calibrations ensures that the values recorded when a patient's blood is analyzed will be correct. It is imperative that these measurements are correct, as changes in patient care will be made based on these values.

Quality Control of an Oxygen Analyzer

Oxygen analyzers should be calibrated prior to each use. Although all analyzers are slightly different, a menu option can place the analyzer in calibration mode. The analyzer will then ask to calibrate to room air and should read 21% when complete. Then the analyzer will ask to analyze to 100%. The analyzer probe should be placed in a container with a 100% oxygen source to ensure that it reads 100%. Once complete, the analyzers should be returned to normal operation mode and staff can be confident that they are analyzing correctly. In addition, prior to any use, the analyzer battery should be checked to ensure that the battery life is adequate for the required task.

Initiation and Modification of Interventions

Maintain a Patent Airway Including the Care of Artificial Airways

Vocally Communicating with a Tracheostomy Tube in Place

Placement of a tracheostomy tube can be done for many reasons, the most common of which is temporary airway placement. This is done when a patient is unable to wean from mechanical ventilation in the desired time. Encouraging communication with a tracheostomy can help instill a feeling of normalcy, which can aid in the psychological improvement of the patient. A tracheostomy is placed in the trachea below the level of the vocal cords. Since speech is produced when airflow is directed over vibrating cords, exhaled air must be redirected. If the patient is able to, he can simply occlude the trach with a finger during exhalation when speaking. If the patient is unable, a speaking valve can be placed, which allows the patient to inhale through the tracheostomy but directs air around the trach through the upper airway during exhalation.

Tracheostomy Care

Tracheostomy care should be performed twice a day to keep the stoma site clean and prevent airway obstruction and infection. Sterile water, cotton-tipped applicators, gauze, and, if needed, isopropyl alcohol should be available for cleaning. Ensure that a manual resuscitator bag and mask, as well as back-up trachs, are available before starting in case of accidental dislodgement. Clean the inner cannula if reusable or replace if disposable. Clean the trach flanges and remove all dried secretions. Clean under the flanges up to the stoma site and assess for any breakdown or infection. Assess trach ties and change if dirty or moist. Inspect the neck for signs of breakdown or redness. If needed, place a pre-cut gauze under the trach flanges to help absorb secretions and provide padding for the skin.

Assessment Criteria for Determining Readiness for Extubation

A patient should be fully assessed prior to removing the endotracheal tube to ensure patient safety and readiness. First, sedation should be minimized or stopped so that there is no interference with the patient's respiratory drive. When it is certain that the patient is sufficiently awake, a spontaneous breathing trial should be performed. At the end of the trial, the patient should be assessed to make sure there has been no substantial change in work of breathing, vital signs, or blood gas values. The patient should have a gag and cough reflex test to ensure he will be able to protect his airway when extubated. Ideally, the patient should be able to follow commands, but this is not required for those presenting with head trauma or neurological insult, such as stroke.

Types of Cuffs Available on Tracheostomy Tubes

There are three main types of tracheostomy tube cuffs, benefiting different types of patients. The first is the standard air cuff. This is the most common type of cuff and is an excellent tool if the patient requires mechanical ventilation, especially high pressures and high PEEP. The pressure should be maintained below 25cm H_2O to minimize risk of damage to the tracheal wall. With air cuffs, the pressure measured through the pilot balloon is equal to the pressure exerted on the tracheal wall. The water cuff is a common cuff used in the pediatric population, although it is also available in adult-sized trachs. The water cuff allows for even distribution of pressure on the tracheal wall and is stable for a longer period of time than air cuffs. Water cuffs do not work well when high pressures or high PEEP is required. Fome cuffs do not need to be inflated, as they self-inflate when they are inserted and the syringe is removed. This type of trach can be used for those on long-term ventilation, but since the cuffs cannot remain deflated long-term, they are not ideal for patients capable of speaking and should never be used with a speaking valve.

Proper Humidification in Patients with Artificial Airways

A normal anatomical airway is designed to filter, heat, and humidify air during inhalation so that by the time air enters the lungs it is 100% saturated and at body temperature. When any artificial airway is placed or the normal airway is diverted, compensation for this warming and humidification must take place to keep secretions manageable and minimize risk of infection. Without humidification, the mucociliary clearance function is severely diminished. Secretions become excessive and thick as they become overwhelmed with debris. The thick mucus becomes more difficult to expectorate, leading to increased chances of infection and pneumonia. Patients with long-term airway diversion, such as those with a tracheostomy or laryngectomy, need to be educated prior to discharge on the importance of humidification and methods to achieve this.

Exchanging a Tracheostomy Tube

Exchanging a tracheostomy tube should be done routinely, based on manufacturer recommendations. The first step is to gather all necessary equipment, which may include: the new trach that will be placed, a trach one size smaller on standby, suction equipment, oxygen/manual resuscitator, new trach ties/securement device, lubrication, sterile water, and gloves. Once the new trach is prepared for insertion, suction the airway if needed. Then remove the old trach ties. When ready, the patient should take a deep breath, if able, and the old tube should be removed. The new tube should be inserted as quickly as possible. Once inserted, remove the obturator from the trach and place an inner cannula if needed. Assessment should be done to ensure the trach is in proper position, including breath sounds and end tidal CO_2, if available. Once placement is confirmed, secure with new trach ties.

Function of a Double Lumen Airway

Double lumen endotracheal tubes are an invasive airway designed to ventilate the left and right lungs independently of each other. Although often used in the operating room for thoracic surgeries to ventilate one lung while the other is undergoing a procedure, they can also be used at the bedside in the intensive care unit for independent lung ventilation. The tube is made up of two lumens, one shorter than the other. The end of the tube is slightly curved. The curved side can be placed in the either the right or left mainstem bronchus, while the shorter tube opening remains in the trachea, directed toward the opposite lung. For example, the curved tip may be placed in the right mainstem while the side opening is pointed toward the left mainstem bronchus. This independent lung ventilation allows for unique ventilation of each lung if there is damage to one but not the other.

Assessments to Perform and Document Following an Extubation

Following an extubation, it is important to properly document patient assessment to show whether the patient tolerated the extubation or if the patient will need additional interventions (high-flow nasal cannula, BiPAP, reintubation). First, a timeout with the team should be performed to ensure that the extubation is occurring on the right patient at the right time. There should be a physician order or appropriate protocol that is followed when extubating a patient. Extubation documentation should include the following data for complete documentation: pre and post heart rate, respiratory, SpO_2, and breath sounds; patient tolerance of procedure; any adverse reactions, even if transient, that may have occurred; what the patient was extubated to (nasal cannula, aerosol mask, room air); the presence or absence of stridor; and any other pertinent data that may be useful for the next providers.

Indications and Contraindications for an Oropharyngeal Airway

Oropharyngeal airways are useful airway adjuncts to remove or diminish airway obstruction by the tongue. An absolute contraindication to an oral airway is consciousness. If the patient is awake or has an intact gag reflex, the patient may vomit with insertion and cause aspiration. Other relative contraindications include recent oral surgery and oral trauma or profuse bleeding. Indication for insertion of an oral airway is to open the mouth and use a bag-valve-mask device to remove the tongue that is causing an obstruction from the airway during manual ventilation. It is also important that the proper size of oropharyngeal airway is used. If the oropharyngeal airway is too large, it may block the airway itself and cause an obstruction. If it is too small, it will not be able to keep the tongue from falling back, and may actually push the tongue further back into the pharynx. The oropharyngeal airway should be measured from the center of the mouth to the angle of the jaw.

Using a Combitube for Airway Management

A Combitube is an emergency airway device, otherwise known as an adjunct or alternate airway, that is designed to be inserted blindly without the use of a laryngoscope. The tube is designed to ventilate a patient if it is inserted into the trachea or esophagus. It is a double lumen tube that has a lower and upper cuff. If inserted into the trachea, the lower cuff is inflated and the tube can be used as an endotracheal tube would be. If it is inserted into the esophagus, the upper cuff is inflated to keep air from escaping back through the mouth and the opening of the lumen directs air into the trachea. A Combitube should not be used long term and should be exchanged for an endotracheal tube if mechanical ventilation is required.

Alteration of the Airway from a Laryngectomy

Laryngectomies are most often performed for laryngeal cancer. Laryngectomy is the surgical removal of the entire larynx. Once the larynx is removed, the trachea is then sutured to the external neck, creating a permanent stoma. This completely separates the upper airway from the lower and the lungs can only be accessed through the stoma. Since the patient is no longer able to be intubated from the nose or mouth, additional equipment should be placed at the bedside. Signage should indicate that the patient has a laryngectomy and that the airway is no longer attached to mouth or nose. An appropriate size trach should be placed in the room so that it can easily be placed in an emergency. A manual resuscitator and pediatric mask should be at the bedside in case mask to stoma resuscitation is required. The patient should also be placed on some type of humidification device while in the hospital.

Speaking Valves

Speaking valves are used for tracheostomized patients and can be used both on and off the ventilator. The speaking valve is a one-way valve that allows the patient to breathe in through the trach, but not to exhale through it. This diverts the exhaled air up and through the vocal cords, allowing the patient to produce speech. Speaking valves are only to be used when the cuff of the tracheostomy tube is completely deflated. In addition, speaking valves can only be used once it is determined that the patient has adequate airflow around the trach to prevent auto-PEEP from occurring. Patients who have been cleared by speech therapy for an oral diet should have the speaking valve in place during eating as it helps to rebalance pressures and resume normal swallowing sensation, which helps prevent aspiration.

Patient Assessments That Should Be Completed Just Prior to Extubation

When a structured method is used for extubation, it minimizes the risk of patient harm and helps to ensure that everything possible has been done to assist the patient in having a successful extubation. First, the patient should demonstrate the ability to breathe on his own. This is routinely done by pressure support trials, T-piece trials, or other modes of ventilation in which a mandatory rate is not set. This will confirm that the patient has an intrinsic respiratory drive to breathe. Also confirm that there are no planned procedures in which an advanced airway will be needed. The patient's oxygen demand should be assessed to ensure that it can be met with noninvasive devices. Blood gases and/or end tidal measurements at the end of any spontaneous breathing trial should show that the patient is able to adequately ventilate (appropriate PCO_2 and pH). A cuff leak should also be present to show that there is no airway swelling or obstruction. Secretions should be of an amount and consistency that can be easily handled by the patient post-extubation to prevent airway obstruction or aspiration. Level of consciousness should be such that the patient has a sufficient cough and gag strength to protect the airway.

Using King Airways

A King airway is a common alternative airway and is classified as a supraglottic airway. The device is designed so that the tip of the tube is placed into the upper portion of the esophagus. The device consists of two cuffs, a proximal and a distal. The distal cuff sits within the upper esophagus and when inflated prevents air from entering the stomach, as well as preventing stomach contents from exiting. The proximal cuff, once inflated, prevents air from escaping into the oropharynx. This two-cuff design allows air to be directed into the lungs during positive pressure ventilation and reduces the chances of aspiration. The King airway is available in seven sizes. The four pediatric sizes are based on weight and are available for patients less than 5kg through 35kg patients. The three adult sizes are based on height and are available from 4 feet to greater than 6 feet. Each size has a color-coded adapter for easy identification.

Contraindications for Using Speaking Valves

Speaking valves can be a useful tool to assist in restoring speech to patients with tracheostomies, but when used improperly they can pose a great risk. Speaking valves should only be used in patients whose tracheostomy tubes are cuffless or have cuffs that completely deflate. In addition, a trial occlusion of the tracheostomy should be performed before placing the speaking valve to ensure adequate airflow around the trach. They should not be used with an inflated cuff or fome cuffs as the patient will not be able to exhale. Speaking valves should never be placed on an endotracheal tube as there will be no airflow around the ETT to produce speech. Speaking valves should never be placed on a patient with a total laryngectomy since the vocal cords have been removed and the airway is now directly attached to the permanent stoma. Speaking valves are also not currently approved for use while sleeping and should only be worn during waking hours.

Diagnosing Ventilator-Associated Incidents/Infections

Diagnosis of ventilator-associated infections is not straightforward and diagnosis criteria may change between institutions. However, there are generally accepted criteria that are evaluated and used in diagnosis. Clinical signs and symptoms, microbiology, blood work, and radiographic data are all examined in making a diagnosis. Clinical signs and symptoms may include hypothermia or hyperthermia and purulent tracheal secretions. Radiographic evaluation of the chest will demonstrate either diffuse or localized infiltrates. Tracheal aspirate cultures may demonstrate moderate or heavy growth of bacteria. A complete blood count may show either leukocytosis or leukopenia, as well as a high number of bands, indicating infection. The patient may also have a decreasing PaO_2/FiO_2 ratio if he begins to develop Acute Respiratory Distress Syndrome (ARDS). An increase in the patient's baseline ventilator settings, including increased PEEP level or FiO_2, can also be indicative of a ventilator-associated infection.

Insertion Technique and Indications for a Nasopharyngeal Airway

Nasopharyngeal airways are considered an airway adjunct. Nasopharyngeal airways can be used in patients in the postoperative period to assist in keeping the upper airway patent, as well as for patients who require repeated nasopharyngeal suctioning. Nasopharyngeal airways should be measured to ensure proper size for the patient. To measure, the nasopharyngeal airway should be held next to the patient's face and should extend from the tip of the nose to the earlobe. This will ensure that it is long enough to reach the back of the throat. Nasopharyngeal airways can be used in a patient who is conscious since it should not stimulate a gag reflex the way an oral airway does. A water-based lubricant should be used to allow smooth insertion and to prevent damage to the sensitive mucosal lining of the nares.

Perform Airway Clearance and Lung Expansion Techniques

Indications for IPV Therapy

Intermittent percussive ventilation is most appropriate for patients with secretions that cannot be cleared with the patient's own cough. This is common in patients recovering from the extended use of sedation or paralytics and for patients with neuromuscular diseases who are unable to initiate a strong cough. IPV therapy can be completed with a mouthpiece or mask, as well as through a tracheostomy. It can also be completed on patients who are intubated and on a ventilator. IPV therapy can last between 5 and 20 minutes per session and is performed 2–4 times daily. Ideally, removal of secretions via spontaneous cough or suctioning should be performed easily post-treatment. IPV therapy can be given simultaneously with nebulized medications, such as hypertonic saline, to further facilitate secretion thinning and removal. The patient should be monitored during therapy, with particular attention to oxygen saturations and heart rate.

Altered Normal Airway Clearance in Patients with Artificial Airways

Altered airways, such as an endotracheal tube, tracheostomy tube, or one in a laryngectomy patient, can alter the patient's ability to clear the airway. The most common cause of impaired airway clearance is improper humidification. Use of inspired air, warmed to body temperature and humidified, is the best method to prevent drying of the airways and increasing thickness of the secretions. In some facilities, cool aerosol is used, but since it lacks the heat normally supplied by the upper airway, it is not as effective. In addition, the administration of certain drugs, especially sedatives and anesthesia medications, can diminish the cough reflex and reduce the ability of the mucociliary escalator to function properly. Intubated patients commonly have underlying pulmonary disease, which can further debilitate airway clearance.

Methods of Assisted Airway Clearance Techniques

Airway clearance devices can be used for both long-term and short-term therapy, depending on the indication. There are many ways both within the hospital and at home to assist a patient in need of bronchial hygiene therapy, and the respiratory therapist should be familiar with five commonly used methods. These techniques are postural drainage, various coughing techniques (such as autogenic drainage or directed coughing), positive airway pressure and positive expiratory pressure devices, frequent turning and moving of the patient, and high-frequency airway oscillation techniques. Many of these techniques can be performed independently for the active patient with chronic disease. Also, multiple therapies may be used on an alternating basis, depending on the state of the disease. For instance, a chronic patient may use positive expiratory pressure devices for normal health and airway oscillation techniques during acute illnesses.

Methods of Performing Airway Suctioning Via an Endotracheal Tube

The two most common methods for suctioning an endotracheal or tracheostomy tube are open catheter and closed catheter. When available, closed catheter suction techniques are preferred as they reduce the need to break the ventilator circuit and can reduce ventilator-associated incidents. This is also a safer method for the healthcare providers as it limits the exposure to bodily fluids. A closed catheter allows for reuse of a single catheter that stays connected to the ventilator circuit and enclosed in a protective plastic sheath. It is changed as needed or per institutional protocol. The use of an open suction catheter requires a new, sterile catheter with each suction attempt and requires that the ventilator circuit be disconnected with each pass into the airway. This method can make the patient more prone to desaturation events and should be avoided, if possible, in patients requiring high PEEP levels.

Using Postural Drainage in Combination with Chest Physiotherapy

Postural drainage involves helping the patient change position during chest physiotherapy so that gravity can assist with removal of secretions from the lungs. It is commonly used in conjunction with manual chest physiotherapy in patients with cystic fibrosis and bronchiectasis. There are 12 possible positions for a patient that can help facilitate the drainage of secretions. The lung segment in focus should be placed in a position superior to the mainstem bronchus of each lung. For example, if the right upper lobe is receiving therapy, the patient should be in an upright position so that as the secretions are loosened they are able to drain downward to the main bronchus to be coughed up and removed. If the lower lung segment is receiving therapy, the patient should be placed in head-down position so that the lower lobe is above the bronchus and secretions will be able to drain down and be coughed up by the patient. The reason for using postural drainage in conjunction with chest physiotherapy is that secretions will be more easily moved to the large airways where they can be removed by the patient's coughing.

Nasotracheal Suctioning

Nasotracheal suctioning is used for patients who have excessive secretions in the nasopharynx and are unable to effectively remove them, either because of a weak cough or the absence of an adequate cough reflex. It is important to perform the procedure without introducing foreign bacteria into the airway. Proper hand hygiene should be performed prior to opening a new, sterile suction catheter. Once the package is opened, sterile gloves should be donned before touching the catheter. A water-based lubricant should be used to prevent damaging the delicate mucosa in the nasal passages. Once lubricated, the catheter should be gently inserted into the nare. The suction catheter is then slowly advanced into the nasopharynx. Suction should only be applied when removing the catheter from the airway. Suction should not be applied for more than 10 seconds to prevent desaturation. Total time in the airway should not exceed 20 seconds.

Side Effects of Performing Airway Clearance Techniques

As with any respiratory therapy administration, patients receiving airway clearance therapy should be monitored closely for adverse reactions and side effects. The most common complication is transient hypoxemia due to the redistribution of secretions within the lung segments and the changes in the ventilation/perfusion ratio as additional lung segments are cleared. If the patient is receiving more invasive therapies such as suctioning, intermittent percussive therapy, and cough assist, it is especially important to watch for this complication. Increased intracranial pressure can occur due to stimulation of the cough reflex, and postural drainage techniques and aggressive airway clearance should be used with caution in patients at risk for elevated intracranial pressures. Vomiting and aspiration are a risk for patients who have recently had food or who are on continuous tube feeding. For those receiving nutrition via a nasogastric or percutaneous tube, feedings should be paused prior to initiation of therapy. Bronchospasm can occur due to forceful coughing and irritation of the airways, especially if inhaled mucolytics are delivered, and a bronchodilator can be used in conjunction with therapy if this is a concern. Less common but severe side effects can include pulmonary hemorrhage, hypotension, and arrhythmias.

Determining the Best Bronchial Hygiene Method

Multiple factors should be considered when determining the most appropriate method of bronchial hygiene therapy. First, it should be determined if the patient is able to assist with the procedure. For most patients, chest physiotherapy, either by hand or with the use of a vest machine, can help loosen secretions. If the patient is unable to assist in the process or has a weak cough reflex, a more invasive method may be needed, such as intermittent percussive ventilation or mechanical insufflation-exsufflation with nasopharyngeal suctioning. Physical limits of the patient should also be considered. The patient should be stable enough to tolerate a full therapy session. In addition, some patients are unable to be turned or to stay in certain positions, which limits the use of postural drainage. The therapist's ability should also be taken into account. If a therapist is unable to perform or uncomfortable with certain techniques and additional help is unavailable, a different approach may be necessary.

Performing Airway Clearance in the Post-Acute or Home Setting

Many of the techniques used in the acute care setting can be transferred to the home setting with proper education of the patient and family. Manual percussive, high-frequency chest wall oscillation, positive expiratory pressure and positive airway pressure therapies, and a cough assist device can all be used for chronic patients at home. The biggest obstacle to certain devices in the home, such as intermittent percussive ventilation therapy, is the lack of high-pressure, 50 psi adaptations in the home setting. Patients who can perform therapy without assistance are set up with chest vest therapy or positive expiratory pressure therapy to perform up to four times a day as indicated by the state of their disease. Patients unable to participate in therapy and who require assistance are prescribed chest vest therapy, manual percussion, or cough assist devices.

Indications for Using a Cough Assist Device

Cough assist devices, or mechanical insufflator-exsufflator devices, are used for patients who cannot produce sufficient force to cough up secretions and foreign objects from the airway. This could be due to overall weakness or debilitation or quadriplegia. The majority of patients who require this type of airway clearance have paralysis or weakened muscles due to neuromuscular disorders. A mechanical insufflator-exsufflator device assists the patient during the inspiratory phase by forcing air into the lungs to provide a larger tidal volume and then removes secretions by switching to a negative pressure phase, sucking air and secretions from the airway. Cough assist therapy is routinely done in "sets" of about five breath cycles, followed by suctioning to remove secretions. Each therapy session consists of 3–5 sets of breaths and is completed 2–4 times a day as indicated by the disease process.

Using an Incentive Spirometer

Incentive spirometers assist the patient in taking deep inspirations and are primarily used in the postoperative phase, when patients are immobile. They can also be a monitoring tool to document and trend the patient's inspiratory volume and to determine whether additional lung expansion therapies are indicated. The patient should be instructed to fully exhale prior to beginning. The patient should then seal his lips around the incentive spirometer mouthpiece and begin a slow, full inhale. The small indicator on the side of the device ensures that the patient is not breathing too slowly or too quickly. The patient should raise the incentive spirometer as high as possible. The patient should also be advised to take a break between each breath to avoid hyperventilation or dizziness, and that coughing may be stimulated by the large breath.

Indications for Bronchial Hygiene Therapy

The respiratory assessment of a patient receiving any respiratory therapy intervention should include assessment for the need for bronchial hygiene therapy. Review of the patient's chart will identify any history of pulmonary disease, recent surgeries, or difficulty with secretion removal. The patient should be assessed for muscle strength, amount of sputum being produced, breath sounds, vital signs, and cough effectiveness. Indications for bronchial hygiene therapy include thick, retained secretions; ineffective cough; atelectasis as seen on chest x-ray or computed tomography; underlying pulmonary disorders with increased secretions (such as cystic fibrosis, pulmonary fibrosis, and interstitial lung disease); postoperative patients with weakened cough due to medications or surgical site pain; and patients who are immobile, either at baseline or due to the current medical or surgical issue. The respiratory therapist should evaluate and recommend an appropriate bronchial hygiene regimen as needed for the individual patient.

Support Oxygenation and Ventilation

Goals of Oxygen Therapy

The goal of oxygen therapy goes beyond just increasing the pulse oximetry reading or PaO_2 value on a blood gas. Acute hypoxemia can cause tachypnea, tachycardia, dyspnea, cyanosis, alterations in blood pressure, altered mental status, headaches, blurred vision, loss of consciousness, and eventually coma or cardiac arrest. Eventually, tissues and organs will not receive the oxygen necessary for metabolic functions, causing tissue damage and organ failure. Oxygen therapy can prevent progression of symptoms and reverse symptoms of hypoxemia. Cardiopulmonary workload is also increased as oxygen delivery to cardiac muscle decreases. Decreased oxygen supply can also lead to pulmonary vasoconstriction and hypertension, causing more hypoxia and workload on the heart. Oxygen therapy can help reverse acute pulmonary hypertension and decrease the workload on the heart. Oxygen therapy can also help with symptoms related to chronic lung diseases such as COPD, emphysema, chronic interstitial lung disease, and pulmonary fibrosis.

Oxygen Toxicity Leads to Worsening Hypoxemia

Although respiratory therapists are usually concerned with delivering enough oxygen, excessive amounts of oxygen can be just as dangerous. The longer a patient is exposed to increased oxygen, the more damage will occur. Damage to the capillaries can lead to interstitial edema. This enlarging of the alveolar-capillary membrane decreases the ability of oxygen to cross from the lungs into the capillaries. Eventually, damage to the alveoli will occur, followed by a decrease in tidal volume and lung capacity. Shunting will increase throughout the lungs, decreasing the ability both to ventilate and oxygenate the patient. This process encourages providers to increase oxygen delivery to increase oxygenation, which only increases damage, perpetuating a deadly cycle. The damage can be seen on x-ray as patchy, fluffy infiltrates, similar to what can be seen in pneumonia or pulmonary edema.

Low-Flow Vs. High-Flow Oxygen Delivery Systems

Low-flow and high-flow systems are not dependent on the set flow; they are determined by how much of the patient's demand is being met with a fixed concentration of oxygen delivery. With low-flow systems, the oxygen delivery flow does not meet the patient's full demand and the FiO_2 delivered will be variable. Although it will provide some of the flow demand, the patient also needs to breathe in surrounding air to meet the full demand. Examples of low-flow devices include nasal cannula, reservoir cannula, simple masks, and partial and non-rebreathing masks. High-flow delivery systems are designed to meet the patient's full inspiratory demand and provide a fixed FiO_2. Examples of high-flow devices include air-entrainment masks, air-entrainment nebulizers, and high-flow, high-humidity nasal cannula systems.

Types of Hemoglobin and Effects on Oxygenation

The presence of abnormal hemoglobin can change how oxygen binds to the hemoglobin in the respiratory capillaries, as well as how oxygen is released from the hemoglobin in the tissues. Sickle hemoglobin (HbS) is the type of abnormal hemoglobin seen in patients with sickle cell disease. The abnormal shape of the hemoglobin (sickle, or C-shaped) can cause the red blood cell to become hard and hemolysis can occur. As additional red blood cells harden and clump together, clots can form, leading to anemia and hypoxemia. Methemoglobin (metHb) occurs when the normal heme complex becomes oxidized, preventing iron from attaching to oxygen. This most commonly occurs with excessive doses of oxidizing medications such as inhaled nitric oxide or nitroglycerin use. Carboxyhemoglobin (HbCO) occurs as a result of inhaling carbon monoxide. Carbon monoxide has a higher affinity for hemoglobin than oxygen, making attaching easier and releasing more difficult. Once HbCO is formed, that hemoglobin molecule is unable to carry oxygen until it is released. Finally, fetal hemoglobin, which is normal in the fetus and children up to 1 year of age, also has a higher affinity for oxygen than adult hemoglobin. This causes fetal hemoglobin to resist releasing oxygen to the tissues.

Effects of Ventilation on Acute Increases in Intracranial Pressure

When patients present with traumatic brain injury, an important aspect of recovery is ensuring that the patient's intracranial pressures stay in a safe range to promote healing and prevent further damage. When intracranial pressure increases, it can cause further damage to brain tissues, leading to further deterioration of brain function. When an acute rise in intracranial pressure occurs, the respiratory therapist can assist by providing appropriate ventilation strategies. $PaCO_2$ levels can greatly affect intracranial pressure through vasodilation or vasoconstriction. As $PaCO_2$ decreases, vasoconstriction increases. This limits excess blood flow to brain, and therefore assists in reducing intracranial pressure. Maintaining $PaCO_2$ between 30 and 35 mm Hg limits excess blood flow, but still supplies enough of the oxygen needed for recovery. When there is an acute increase in pressure, short-term hyperventilation can help decrease intracranial pressure until additional therapies can be initiated.

Oxygenation Index

Oxygenation index is determined by multiplying the FiO_2 by the mean airway pressure and dividing by the PaO_2. The lower the oxygenation index, the more efficiently the body can uptake and use oxygen in the tissues. There are differing values of what is considered normal, but an oxygenation index greater than 15 is a concern for lung disease that is inhibiting oxygenation, and a value greater than 20 is a concern for severe lung disease causing tissue hypoxia. If the patient has an oxygenation index greater than 40, extracorporeal membrane oxygenation (ECMO) should be considered since the lungs cannot provide adequate oxygen delivery to the tissues and organs of the body. The risk of morbidity and mortality greatly increase with oxygen index values over 40.

Monitoring Capnometry

Capnometry is the continuous monitoring of exhaled carbon dioxide. Monitoring of capnographic measurements can be done with either a sidestream device or a mainstream device. A sidestream device pulls a volume of air from the ventilator circuit to analyze the results. A mainstream device is placed in line with the circuit and measures the CO_2 directly in the circuit. Capnometry can be used for a variety of reasons in the mechanically ventilated patient, including CO_2 trending to reduce the number of frequent arterial blood draws, assessing the severity of pulmonary disease, ensuring tracheal intubation as opposed to esophageal intubation, and assuring a patent airway during mechanical ventilation. In addition, capnometry can be used in non-intubated patients, especially when giving conscious sedation to monitor the patient's breathing patterns. When using in line with mechanical ventilation, it is important to remember that it does add additional dead space, which may or may not be clinically significant.

Automatic Tube Compensation

Automatic tube compensation is an option on certain models of mechanical ventilators to assist the patient during spontaneous breaths by overcoming the resistance to the tube. When performing the initial setup, the patient category (neo, ped, adult) is chosen, along with the inner diameter of the airway being used (endotracheal tube size). When activated, automatic tube compensation will adjust the levels of pressure support to overcome the expected work of breathing due to the endotracheal tube. The percentage of the work of breathing can be adjusted, but at 100%, it is theorized that the work of breathing would be equal to breathing without the tube. Spontaneous breathing trials can be performed with the use of automatic tube compensation, rather than setting pressure support levels, to determine if the patient has the necessary muscle strength to be successfully extubated.

Advantages and Disadvantages of Square and Decelerating Waveforms

Square waveforms, also known as constant flow waveforms, tend to require the shortest inspiratory time to deliver a set volume, but require the highest inspiratory pressures. The mean airway pressure is lower than other available waveforms. Decelerating waveforms require a longer inspiratory time to deliver a set volume, but they result in lower peak inspiratory pressure. The overall mean airway pressure tends to be higher. Decelerating waveforms are the preferred waveform for many practitioners due to the fact that they most resemble the natural inspiratory process, increasing patient ventilator synchrony. A decelerating waveform also provides increased oxygenation due to the increased mean airway pressure, and achieves this with a lower peak inspiratory pressure. The downfalls of the decelerating waveform include the chance of increased intracranial pressure and decreased cardiac output due to increased mean airway pressures, as well as the possibility of auto-PEEP due to the longer inspiratory time and shorter expiratory time.

Inclusion and Exclusion Criteria for Noninvasive Ventilation

The use of noninvasive ventilation has dramatically reduced the need for intubation in patients presenting with type II respiratory failure, especially those with chronic respiratory disorders such as COPD. The respiratory therapist must understand when and when not to use noninvasive ventilation, based on the patient's presenting symptoms. Acute hypercapnic respiratory failure is defined as a pH of less than 7.35 and a $PaCO_2$ of greater than 65 mm Hg and the patient should be considered for noninvasive ventilation. Exclusion criteria include an inability to protect one's airway, impending respiratory arrest, untreated pneumothorax, facial injuries that would interfere with mask placement, and metabolic acidosis. Also, patients who present with vomiting, altered mental status, or inability to control secretions should be discussed prior to initiation to ensure that the risks do not outweigh the benefits.

P/F Ratio

P/F ratio is the ratio of the patient's PaO_2 and FiO_2. It is an equation that gives a numerical representation of the patient's ability to oxygenate. The higher the P/F ratio, the better the patient is exchanging gases. A normal P/F ratio is 500. A P/F ratio of less than 300 indicates the presence of acute lung injury (ALI). A P/F ratio of 200 or less is severe and indicates the patient is suffering from Acute Respiratory Distress Syndrome (ARDS). For many ECMO centers, a P/F ratio of less than 150 indicates placement on extracorporeal membrane oxygenation. The respiratory therapist should calculate the P/F ratio with each arterial blood gas, as trending can help in early identification of patients with worsening lung disease.

Hysteresis in Regard to the Pressure-Volume Loop in Ventilation

The pressure-volume loop on the ventilator shows how lung compliance changes as volume changes. The shape of the loop can help the respiratory therapist identify compliance issues in the lungs, such as underinflation, overdistension and optimal compliance. "Beaking" at the top of the loop, the upper inflection point, indicates lung overdistension, in which the alveoli are being stretched beyond the optimal distension point, whereas the lower inflection point can help determine alveoli critical opening pressure. When the lower inflection point is well rounded without beaking, it indicates an ideal PEEP level. At this PEEP setting, the alveoli can remain open at the end of exhalation with adequate distension and without collapse. Pressure-volume loops should be assessed with each ventilator check as lung compliance can change quickly and settings may need to be adjusted.

Factors That Can Diminish a Patient's Respiratory Drive

Patients in the acute and critical care setting need to be watched carefully for respiratory depression, or a decrease in respiratory drive. Respiratory depression can be caused by a variety of interventions unrelated to the respiratory system. Increased CO_2 will increase a patient's respiratory drive, but only to a critical point. Once CO_2 levels reach this critical level, it will result in respiratory depression. In addition, if CO_2 is critically low, patients will experience respiratory depression or respiratory arrest as there is no chemical drive to breathe. Pain medications and narcotics can lead to respiratory depression, and even respiratory arrest, if doses are too high. Stroke, swelling, shear injuries, and trauma to the brainstem can cause respiratory depression, as the respiratory control center is located in the brainstem. Neuromuscular diseases, obesity, sleep apnea, and hypoventilation syndrome also increase the risk of respiratory depression.

Issues That Can Increase a Patient's Respiratory Workload

Respiratory workload can be impacted by both internal and external factors. Respiratory workload can be defined as the amount of work the patient must overcome in order to breathe effectively for gas exchange. Diseases such as emphysema cause air trapping and overdistension of the lungs to the point that inhaling becomes difficult because the lungs are so full. Morbid obesity causes pressure on the lungs to the point that inhaling becomes difficult as the diaphragms become more and more elevated. Any disorder or disease that affects the respiratory muscles or chest wall also increases respiratory workload as the patient must now overcome these forces. Upper airway obstructions and swelling create the need for higher inspiratory work to overcome these obstacles. For intubated patients, if artificial airways are too small, resistance to airflow is increased.

Effect of the Oxyhemoglobin Disassociation Curve on Oxygenation

The oxyhemoglobin disassociation curve is used to estimate blood oxygen tension at specific levels of hemoglobin saturation percentage. Shifting of the curve to the right or left affects how much oxygen is available for use, compared to oxygen demand. Factors that shift the curve to the left cause a lower oxygen tension at the same hemoglobin saturation percentage. Shifts in the curve to the right cause increased levels of oxygen tension at the same level of hemoglobin saturation. Factors that can cause the curve to shift left (lower oxygen levels) include alkalosis, hypothermia, decreased PCO_2, low levels of 2,3-DPG, carboxyhemoglobin, and methemoglobin. Factors that can cause the curve to shift to the right (higher oxygen levels) include acidosis, increased PCO_2, hyperthermia, abnormal hemoglobin, and high levels of 2,3-DPG. Understanding how these factors affect oxygenation levels is important for respiratory management of acutely ill patients.

Mechanism Behind High-Flow Nasal Cannulas

A high-flow nasal cannula is a high-flow oxygen device, meaning that it can meet or exceed the patient's inspiratory demand with a fixed FiO_2. High-flow nasal cannulas have been used in the neonatal and pediatric population for many years as an alternative to CPAP. The high-flows that can be generated with 100% heated and humidified air can expand the lungs nearly as well as CPAP in most children, but in an apparatus that is often more tolerated than CPAP masks or nasal prongs. In recent years, the utility of high-flow nasal cannulas has been seen in the adult population, especially for patients in acute COPD exacerbation, as an alternative to BiPAP. In adults, flows of up to 60L/min can be achieved. High-flow nasal cannulas are able to remove CO_2 in anatomic dead space, increasing ventilation for the patient. The high-flows are able to create end expiratory pressure, helping to recruit collapsed alveoli and increase lung volumes.

Indications for Placement of a Tracheostomy Tube

Tracheostomy tubes can be placed for a variety of reasons, the most common of which are long-term intubation and mechanical ventilation. Long-term intubation can cause severe damage to the upper airway and vocal cords, so tracheostomy is performed to facilitate long-term ventilator weaning in patients who are unable to be extubated. In addition to long-term mechanical ventilation, tracheostomy can be performed for severe sleep apnea in which CPAP/BiPAP via mask is not sufficient. Airway abnormalities, such as tracheomalacia or tumors compressing the airway, may require tracheostomy until a long-term surgical solution can be determined. Urgent tracheostomies can be performed when intubation is not possible. It is important to remember that not all tracheostomy patients will require mechanical ventilation, as some only need to ensure a patent upper airway.

Advantages and Disadvantages in Using High-Frequency Oscillatory Ventilation

High-frequency oscillatory ventilation is usually implemented when conventional ventilation is not adequately oxygenating the patient. Although considered a "gentler" form of mechanical ventilation, it can be intimidating for family and staff who are not familiar with its use. High-frequency oscillatory ventilation works by expanding the lungs to a set mean airway pressure and provides both active inhalation and active exhalation without the repeated expansion and deflation required by each breath on a conventional ventilator. High-frequency oscillatory ventilation can provide higher mean airway pressures than conventional ventilation, increasing oxygenation since it does not cause the damage that traditional lung expansion does. However, patients are at risk for pneumothorax and hypotension, especially during the initiation phase as mean airway pressure increases. The benefits of high frequency oscillatory ventilation in the adult population are still being studied, but it has been shown to be beneficial in the neonatal and pediatric populations.

Administer Medications and Specialty Gases

Indications and Mechanism of Action for Inhaled Nitric Oxide

Nitric oxide is a colorless, odorless gas delivered via inhalation. It is FDA approved for use in term and near-term neonates (>35 weeks) with persistent pulmonary hypertension of the newborn (PPHN). It has recently been used off label in the pediatric and adult populations when conventional methods of increasing oxygen were not successful. Nitric oxide is a selective pulmonary vasodilator with a short half-life (6 seconds), so it has minimal impact outside the pulmonary vasculature. It acts on the smooth muscle of the pulmonary vasculature to relax the muscles, dilating blood vessels and lowering pulmonary blood pressure. Two tanks should always be available in case of malfunction, as the half-life is so short. Abrupt removal of nitric oxide can cause severe rebound pulmonary hypertension that can be life-threatening.

Classes of Medications for Aerosol Delivery

There are seven distinct classes of medications that can be aerosolized for delivery via inhalation. Adrenergic bronchodilators are the most common aerosolized medication and include racemic epinephrine, albuterol, levalbuterol, and salmeterol, among others. Anticholinergic bronchodilators, such as ipratropium bromide, are often given in conjunction with adrenergic medications. Mucoactive, or mucus controlling, medications are delivered to assist in airway clearance and include acetylcysteine, dornase alfa, and hypertonic saline. Inhaled corticosteroids are routinely given for long-term management of respiratory disorders and include budesonide in the aerosolized form. Nonsteroidal antiasthmatic medications include cromolyn sodium in the aerosolized form. Aerosolized anti-infectives are routinely used to deliver antibiotics and antiretrovirals directly to the lungs and include pentamidine, ribavirin, tobramycin, and aztreonam. Finally, inhaled pulmonary vasodilators, such as iloprost and treprostinil, are delivered via the aerosolized route.

Indications for Inhaled Specialty Gases (NO, HeO_2, N)

There are a variety of specialty gases available to the respiratory therapist for treatment and symptom management of patients. Inhaled nitric oxide is an inhaled pulmonary vasodilator used for newborns with persistent pulmonary hypertension and meconium aspiration syndrome. Heliox is a combination of helium and oxygen. The lightweight helium is able to carry oxygen past obstructive areas and can be especially helpful for patients with upper airway swelling and stridor, and for patients with lower airway restriction, such as acute asthma exacerbation. When delivered with aerosolized medications, it can improve deposition into the lower airways. Helium/oxygen mixtures are usually described as 80/20, 70/30, or 60/40. At less than 60% helium, the mixture loses its beneficial lightweight characteristic. Nitrogen is a gas that can be given to patients with congenital cardiac defects that are causing pulmonary overcirculation. Adding nitrogen lowers the overall FiO_2, which allows for delivery of subatmospheric oxygen levels, usually in the range of 17% to 20%. This assists with pulmonary vasoconstriction to reduce blood flow to the lungs until a surgical intervention can be performed.

Scenario

Patients with chronic respiratory disorders and frequent respiratory infections require rigorous pulmonary interventions that may consist of airway clearance, mucolytics, antibiotics, bronchodilators, and corticosteroids. Explain the order interventions should be administered and why.

> The order in which medications are delivered can alter their efficacy, especially in patients with chronic disorders such as cystic fibrosis. The first medication should be the bronchodilator. It will help relax and open up the airways, preparing them for rest of the medications. The second medication should be mucolytics to help break up the secretions, making them easier to cough out. Once the mucolytics have been given, airway clearance, such as chest physiotherapy or PEP device, should be completed to remove as many of the secretions as possible before the remaining medications are delivered. Corticosteroids are the next medication given to help decrease airway inflammation. Antibiotics are always delivered last, once the airways are open and cleared, so that they can remain in the airways as long as possible to kill infection.

Mechanism of Action of Various Inhaled Medication Classifications

Adrenergic medications are bronchodilators that affect alpha-receptors, beta-1 receptors, and beta-2 receptors. The stimulation of beta-2 receptors creates bronchodilation through relaxation of the bronchial smooth muscles and stimulation of mucociliary clearance ability. Anticholinergic bronchodilators reduce airflow obstruction by blocking muscarinic receptors, preventing cholinergic bronchoconstriction. The two currently approved mucus-controlling agents are N-Acetylcysteine (10% and 20%) and Dornase Alpha. N-Acetylcysteine acts by breaking the disulfide bond in the mucus, causing a thinning of gel-like secretions and allowing the patient to expectorate the secretions much more easily. Dornase Alpha is an enzyme that thins secretions caused by infections in patients with cystic fibrosis. Dornase Alpha attacks the DNA strands that make the sputum thick, allowing the patient to expectorate it when it thins.

Possible Side Effects of Aerosolized Corticosteroids

Corticosteroids are hormones that have an anti-inflammatory property within the body. When nebulized and inhaled, they provide anti-inflammatory therapy for long-term maintenance for patients with chronic respiratory disorders such as COPD and asthma. Since corticosteroids used for respiratory disease are inhaled, they do not have the same systemic side effects that oral or intravenous delivery of steroids can have. However, this does not mean that they cannot produce systemic side effects or that they are benign. The most common side effects are local, causing issues in the respiratory tract, including alterations in voice as the medication is inhaled and comes in contact with the vocal cords, fungal infections in the mouth (oral thrush) when not rinsed properly after use, and bronchoconstriction in some patients. Long-term use can have systemic side effects, such as bone weakening and adrenal insufficiency.

Possible Adverse Reactions of Inhaled Nitric Oxide

Nitric oxide is frequently used in neonates with persistent pulmonary hypertension and certain congenital cardiac defects. However, if the inhaled nitric oxide is delivered to a newborn who is considered dependent on a right to left shunt for adequate blood flow, it can cause rapid dilation of pulmonary vessels and a decrease in pulmonary blood pressure. When pulmonary blood pressure decreases, patients can lose that right to left shunt, decreasing peripheral perfusion and therefore end organ perfusion. High doses of nitric oxide can also lead to the formation of methemoglobin, preventing hemoglobin from carrying oxygen to the needed organs and tissues of the body. Abrupt discontinuation of nitric oxide therapy can also cause rebound pulmonary hypertension from rapid vasoconstriction of the pulmonary vessels. Care should be taken to wean nitric oxide slowly over hours or days to prevent this from occurring.

Indications and Complications of Hyperbaric Oxygen Treatment

Hyperbaric oxygen therapy is high-level oxygen delivery at high pressures (usually between 1 and 3 atm). The goal of hyperbaric therapy is hyperoxia. The high-pressure delivery fully saturates the plasma with oxygen, allowing for maximal tissue uptake. Indications for hyperbaric oxygen therapy are numerous, but the most common include treatment for decompression sickness, necrotizing infections in the tissues, treatment of wounds resulting from decreased perfusion, and healing of skin grafts after conventional therapies have failed. During hyperbaric therapy, patients must be closely watched, and initiation and discontinuation of the therapy treatment should be performed by a trained provider. Complications of hyperbaric therapy include pneumothorax, gas emboli, ear and sinus pain, and oxygen toxicity. Serious complications can include hypotension, sudden decompression from equipment malfunction, and fire due to the high levels of oxygen.

Ideal Nitric Delivery Systems

Nitric oxide therapy can be a life-saving intervention for many neonatal patients, but the respiratory therapist should take care to ensure proper setup and handling of the delivery system. The delivery system should be able to reliably deliver a set dosage of nitric oxide, given the potential for toxicity of overdose and the need for precise weaning (usually 1 ppm every 6–12 hours) to prevent rebound pulmonary hypertension. The setup should also have a backup delivery option in case of primary delivery failure. Constant monitoring of the delivered dose of nitric oxide, as well as the nitrogen dioxide, is also a crucial part of the system. Alarms should be set to alert the practitioner if the nitric oxide set dose is not being delivered to the patient, if the nitrogen dioxide rises above critical levels within the circuit (usually kept below 2 ppm), and if the delivered FiO_2 is out of the set range. Ideally, the system should include a way to attach a second tank prior to disconnecting the main tank for safer switching, considering the extremely short half-life.

Elements Reducing Aerosol Delivery to the Lungs

The factors that most often reduce aerosol delivery to lungs are human factors or incorrect administration techniques. Patients should be instructed on proper breathing technique to ensure optimal delivery. Patients should refrain from talking during nebulizer therapy. In addition, when giving nebulizers to infants and children, it is important to keep the patient calm and prevent crying or screaming during the therapy. Patients who have a low minute volume or shallow breathing will not be able to take a deep breath to get the medication into the lower airways where it is needed. Artificial airways will also reduce medication delivery as there is an increased chance of deposition on the artificial airway rather than in the lower airways. Patients with severe airway obstruction or small airways, such as children, will also have less deposition as the particles will have difficulty bypassing and depositing into the lower airways.

Aerosolized Antimicrobial Drugs

Some antimicrobial drugs are aerosolized to treat infections within the lungs. One common drug that is administered via aerosol is tobramycin. This antimicrobial can be used to treat lung infections, specifically *Pseudomonas aeruginosa* infections in immunocompromised patients such as those with cystic fibrosis. This drug can also be used for ventilator-associated pneumonia, some forms of bronchiectasis, and some mycobacterial infections; however, the most common use for aerosolized tobramycin is for the treatment of infections secondary to cystic fibrosis. The medication is placed in a small-volume nebulizer, and it is attached to an oxygen flow meter. The flow is dialed in to approximately 8 liters per minute, and the treatment commences. The patient uses either a mask or a mouthpiece and inhales the medication until there is no drug left in the nebulizer cup. This medication is often given alone, not in combination with bronchodilators; however, it can be given immediately after other nebulizer treatments.

Ensure Modifications are Made to the Respiratory Care Plan

Indications and Side Effects of Administering an Inhaled Bronchodilator

Bronchodilators can be divided into two sub groups: short-acting bronchodilators (SABA) and long-acting bronchodilators (LABA). Short-acting bronchodilators are used for acute processes and causes of bronchoconstriction considered to be reversible, such as bronchospasm. This includes exacerbation of chronic diseases, such as asthma, bronchitis, and cystic fibrosis. They can also be used for bronchoconstriction caused by exposure, such as anaphylaxis. Patient assessment will show expiratory and/or inspiratory wheezing, and a prolonged expiratory phase with diminished or absent breath sounds in severe attacks. Long-acting bronchodilators are used for maintaining bronchodilation and for control and prevention of acute processes, such as in asthma, emphysema, and chronic obstructive pulmonary disease. Possible side effects of bronchodilator therapy include tachycardia, decreasing ventilation/perfusion ratio, dizziness, hypokalemia, and relaxation of airways, causing lower airways to collapse (bronchomalacia).

Assessments for Monitoring Effectiveness of a Current Regimen

Patients should be instructed on the use of a peak flow meter to be used at the same time every day to monitor lung function. Arterial blood gases can be done during acute exacerbations of chronic disease, as well as intermittently in a physician's office, to assess baseline CO_2 retention levels. Blood glucose can increase with beta agonist therapy and should be monitored. In addition, potassium may decrease with therapy and should also be monitored. Patients on multiple therapies should be able to describe when to use each medication (daily or rescue) and demonstrate proper use. Pulmonary function tests should be done periodically to assess disease state and baseline lung function. When assessing whether to adjust long-acting therapy, the practitioner should consider the number of emergency room or unscheduled clinic visits and the average number of times the patient uses a rescue inhaler per day/week/month.

Indications to Initiate or Discontinue Lung Expansion Therapy

Lung expansion therapy, or intermittent positive airway pressure, is used as an adjunct therapy when there is evidence of atelectasis or low lung volumes, or when patients are at high risk for either. Postoperative abdominal or thoracic surgery patients are at risk for developing atelectasis due to pain on inspiration from the surgical site. Patients presenting with rib fractures after trauma are also at risk of lung collapse and atelectasis. These patients may benefit from lung expansion therapy 3–4 times a day, in addition to routine incentive spirometry use and ambulation, to prevent atelectasis and resulting infection or pneumonias that can complicate recovery. Lung expansion therapy may also be considered for patients presenting with weakness due to age, infection, or neuromuscular disorders such as myasthenia gravis or Guillain-Barré.

Effects of Prone Patient Positioning on Oxygenation and Ventilation

When a patient remains in a supine position for an extended period of time, especially patients suffering from acute respiratory distress syndrome, lung damage in the dorsal lung regions may occur. This damage increases ventilation/perfusion mismatching and decreases both the oxygenation and ventilation ability of the lungs. When a patient is placed prone, especially early in the disease process, it can relieve pressure on the dorsal areas and allow for movement of retained secretions from this area. When proning a patient with dorsal lung damage secondary to supine positioning, the anterior aspects of the lung that have better aeration are now in the dependent regions, and as perfusion increases in these areas, the ventilation/perfusion mismatch will begin to decrease. This decrease in mismatch and decrease in shunting allows for an increase in both oxygenation and ventilation.

Weaning of Inhaled Nitric Oxide

Nitric oxide is a vascular smooth muscle relaxer that is naturally released by the body in small amounts. When inhaled, it is a potent pulmonary vasodilator that can lower pulmonary pressures with few systemic side effects. When weaning off of inhaled nitric oxide, it must be withdrawn slowly. During delivery, the body's production of nitric oxide decreases. When removed abruptly, the body does not have time to increase its natural production, resulting in rebound pulmonary hypertension. In general, once the patient has stabilized and weaning is begun, nitric oxide is decreased by 5 ppm every 6–12 hours. Once the patient reaches 5 ppm, weaning should continue at 1 ppm every 6–12 hours. Prior to discontinuing, the patient should be preoxygenated to ensure that discontinuation will not cause a decrease in oxygen levels.

Indications and Side Effects of Administering Diuretics for a Patient in Respiratory Distress

A patient in respiratory failure, especially a patient in acute respiratory distress syndrome, may also present with an imbalance of fluid. Fluid management is a major area of concern for patients admitted to the intensive care unit. Fluid management and careful documentation of intake and output can prevent further respiratory problems related to fluid overload. If the patient becomes fluid overloaded, fluid can leak from the pulmonary capillaries and cause fluid to accumulate in and around the lungs, leading to pulmonary vascular congestion and even pulmonary edema. For patients who have a positive fluid balance from fluid resuscitation, administering diuretics can assist the patient in removing excess fluid via urination. However, care should be taken not to over-diurese the patient. In addition to losing too much fluid, other side effects include potassium imbalances (hypo- or hyperkalemia), hyponatremia, muscle cramps, headaches, and increased thirst. Serious side effects include renal failure and heart arrhythmias.

Effects of Positive Pressure Ventilation on Renal Function

Patients who are critically ill and require mechanical ventilation are at risk for other organ system failures. When a patient is on mechanical ventilation, daily weights and close monitoring of intake and output are important to ensure that the body is maintaining an adequate fluid balance. When positive pressure ventilation is administered, the increased intrathoracic pressure can change blood flow dynamics in the chest, leading to a decrease in venous return as blood flows back to the heart, as well as decreased output as blood flow is leaving the chest. As blood pressure decreases, blood flow to the kidneys also decreases, affecting glomerular filtration rate and disrupting sodium and potassium balance. Fluid volume during mechanical ventilation should be carefully monitored, keeping intravascular volume as close to normal as possible to prevent acute kidney injury.

Medications for Acute and Chronic Pulmonary Hypertension

When a patient develops an acute exacerbation or onset of pulmonary hypertension, inhaled medications deliver the quickest onset with the least systemic side effects. Nitric oxide is a gaseous inhaled pulmonary vasodilator that can be set up quickly and can be given in-line with invasive and noninvasive respiratory support. Flolan is a nebulized pulmonary vasodilator given via a continuous nebulizer. Either medication can be used for short-term, immediate intervention of pulmonary hypertension. Long-term, medications can be given via nebulization, intravenous, or oral methods to control symptoms. Prostanoids can be delivered via continuous IV infusion, but can have many adverse side effects. Nebulized medications can be given, but require administration 4–9 times per day. Endothelin-receptor antagonists, such as Bosentan, are another class of medications available that can improve quality of life for patients with PAH. Sildenafil is a phosphodiesterase type 5 inhibitor, which allows for a longer-lasting effect than nitric oxide.

Factors to Assess When Deciding to Discontinue Ventilator Support

The patient should be assessed daily for readiness to wean from the ventilator to ensure that he does not stay intubated longer than necessary. The longer the patient remains intubated, the greater the chance of adverse events, such as infection, pneumonia, or upper airway and vocal cord damage. Assessment for discontinuing the ventilator should include: the initial cause of needing ventilator support should be resolved, FiO_2 of less than or equal to 0.5, PEEP level of 5-8 cm H_2O, an adequate drive to breathe, and adequate respiratory muscle strength. The patient should be under no, or minimal, sedation that could interfere with the ability to breathe independently. Cough and gag reflexes should be intact to ensure that the patient can protect the airway. In addition, the patient should have a forceful enough cough to expectorate foreign matter from the lungs.

Recommending Patient Extubation After a Successful Weaning Trial

Successful weaning trials and successful extubation are two different entities and should be individually assessed. Once a patient has passed a spontaneous breathing trial, the patient should be assessed for ability to maintain the airway. Ideally, when the pilot balloon on the endotracheal tube is deflated, air should be able to leak from around the tube. This ensures that the airway is not edematous and is patent around the endotracheal tube. The patient should have an appropriate cough and gag reflex to ensure that he can effectively clear secretions from the airway. The patient should be off sedation or on minimal sedation that could inhibit the respiratory drive. Ideally, patients should be alert and able to follow commands, although in some cases the care team may opt for extubation even if the patient is not alert, especially if head trauma was the cause of intubation. These patients may be able to maintain their airway, but need extensive rehabilitation. In some cases, a tracheostomy may be needed if there is concern about airway compromise.

Influence of Nebulized Albuterol on Potassium Levels

Catecholamines, such as epinephrine, can cause an increase in the action of the sodium potassium pumps in the cell wall. When activated, potassium from the serum is pumped into the cell while the cell pumps sodium into the serum. Albuterol, a beta 2-adrenergic medication, can act similarly to catecholamines, activating the sodium potassium pump. This decreases the level of potassium in the serum. Low levels of potassium (hypokalemia) can cause muscle weakness, muscle spasms, and cardiac arrhythmias. Although single nebulizers of albuterol are unlikely to have a large enough impact to affect potassium levels, patients on high doses of frequent nebulizers (every 2 hours) or those receiving continuous nebulization of albuterol may benefit from having potassium levels checked intermittently during administration.

Ventilator Setting Changes to Correct an Uncompensated Respiratory Acidosis

Uncompensated respiratory acidosis is characterized by a decrease in pH and an increase in CO_2, with no change in the bicarbonate levels. When the patient is on a ventilator with an uncompensated respiratory acidosis, there are two primary ways of correcting the imbalance. The first way is to increase the set respiratory rate. The higher the CO_2 level, the greater the needed change in respiratory rate. Also, the amount of air exchanged with each breath can be manipulated. If the patient is on a Volume Control mode, the tidal volume can be increased. If the patient is on a Pressure Control mode, an increase in peak pressure will cause a greater volume of air to be displaced, as long as the PEEP is not also adjusted. As with any ventilator changes, be sure to assess the patient after changes are made.

Treatment of Pneumothorax Recommendations

Pneumothorax is the buildup of air within the pleural space around the lung. If left untreated, pneumothorax can result in lung collapse, cardiac compression, and death. Pneumothorax can be caused by trauma to the chest, spontaneous pneumothorax due to underlying lung disease, or spontaneous without underlying lung disease. The first treatment is to place the patient on oxygen. Since the majority of the air within a pneumothorax is nitrogen, placing the patient on high FiO_2 increases the nitrogen gradient, allowing nitrogen to be reabsorbed and slowly decreasing the pneumothorax. Aspiration of the air within the pleural space by inserting a needle through the chest wall between the ribs can also be performed to quickly relieve the pneumothorax. If the pneumothorax is recurrent, a chest tube can be placed to drain the air until it no longer accumulates. Pleurodesis can be performed for patients with recurrent pneumothorax.

Factors Influencing Interventions and Patient Outcome in Near-Drowning

When a patient is brought into the emergency department as a drowning patient, questions should be asked that can impact a patient's long-term outcome:

- Was the submersion witnessed? Witnessed drownings generally have a higher survival rate as resuscitation begins sooner. If the patient was submerged for longer than 10 minutes, the chance of survival with neurological recovery is close to 0%.
- Did the patient lose consciousness? Most drowning victims will lose consciousness after three minutes underwater. The longer the victim remains unconscious, the lower the chances of achieving neurological recovery.
- What was the water temperature? Patients submerged in cold water have a better chance of recovery than those who are submerged in warm water. The colder temperatures lower the core body temp as well as the metabolic and oxygen demand of vital organs.
- Was the water fresh or saltwater? Fresh water has a tendency to carry fewer bacteria that can infest the lungs; however it is still not considered clean water. Fresh water and saltwater also disrupt the body's balance of sodium and other electrolytes, albeit in different ways, so close monitoring is necessary.

Respiratory Intervention Recommendations for Patients Presenting with Burn Injury

A patient presenting with burn injury, especially to the face, upper body, and torso, can be challenging for the respiratory therapist in terms of ventilation. If the airway is considered stable, humidified air can be administered to help soothe the airway and decrease airway inflammation and swelling. If stridor is present because of swelling, nebulized racemic epinephrine can help decrease swelling for a short period of time. IV administration of steroids can assist in decreasing airway swelling as well. If an attempt to stave off intubation is warranted, heliox therapy can be administered to ease breathing work due to swelling of the airways. Airway swelling can occur rapidly in these patients and it is best to intubate patients prophylactically. Intubation should be performed in a controlled environment and access to surgical airways (tracheostomy or cricothyroidotomy) should be available in case an airway cannot be achieved. Once airway swelling occurs, the risk of being unable to intubate increases, and therefore the risk of needing a surgical airway also increases.

Respiratory Disorders Related to Obesity and Recommended Interventions

The number one respiratory concern in obese patients is the development of obstructive sleep apnea. Untreated, sleep apnea can lead to pulmonary hypertension and heart failure. The risk of obstructive sleep apnea increases as the circumference of the neck increases, and men have a greater chance of developing sleep apnea than women. In addition, obesity can lead to obesity hypoventilation syndrome, in which the body retains carbon dioxide, and in some cases lowers the amount of oxygen in the blood. The risk of pneumonia, acute respiratory distress syndrome, and pulmonary embolism are also greater in patients with an elevated body mass index. The mere presence of excess weight around the abdomen and chest cavities can cause a restrictive lung disease since the lungs are not able to expand properly with the additional fat accumulation.

Recommended Interventions for Newborns Presenting with Meconium Aspiration Syndrome

Meconium aspiration syndrome mainly affects postterm newborns (greater than 41 weeks gestation). When possible, prevention is the best strategy by inducing labor prior to 41 weeks and reducing stress to the fetus' environment. Once delivered, the first step is to assess the infant for immediate resuscitative needs (positive pressure ventilation, oxygen, intubation). Once the infant is stabilized, it is important to watch for signs and symptoms of persistent pulmonary hypertension. In severe cases of meconium aspiration syndrome, high-frequency oscillation or high-frequency jet ventilation may be needed to reduce lung injury. Patients with meconium aspiration syndrome can be difficult to ventilate due to the heterogenous lung insult that occurs. Segments of the lung may be underinflated or collapsed, while neighboring segments may be overinflated. Extracorporeal membrane oxygenation may be required if the infant has comorbidities, such as persistent pulmonary hypertension.

Circumstances for Recommending Replacement of an in Situ Endotracheal Tube

Endotracheal tube exchange can be necessitated for a variety of reasons. Unlike other indwelling lines and catheters, routine exchanges or time limits based on infectious reasons alone are not reasons to exchange an endotracheal tube, due to the high risk of being unable to reinsert a new tube and patient decompensation during the procedure. The most common reason to exchange an endotracheal tube is for tube occlusion that cannot be resolved with suctioning. Additional reasons include changing the tube size to either a larger or smaller tube depending on the presence or absence of an air leak and tube malfunction, such as a cuff that will not remain inflated. Less likely reasons include changing the tube type for a surgical procedure (double lumen tube) or changing tube location (nasal to oral or oral to nasal).

Recommended Treatment for a Patient Presenting with Bronchiolitis

Bronchiolitis is inflammation of the airways, usually caused by or following a viral illness. It usually affects children and infants, but can occasionally be the cause of respiratory distress in compromised adults. In most cases, patients will not need to be hospitalized and supportive therapy can be given at home. In cases where hospitalization is necessary, supportive care is the main goal, including oxygen therapy, such as high-flow/high-humidity oxygen to support a patient's work of breathing. IV fluids may need to be administered if the patient's oral intake is insufficient. Patients who become dehydrated may have thicker secretions, increasing the chance of further complications, such as pneumonia or mucus plugging. Tylenol or ibuprofen may be administered for irritability or fever reduction as needed. Patients with preexisting pulmonary conditions, such as bronchopulmonary dysplasia or chronic lung disease, are at higher risk for more severe complications and should be watched closely.

Disease Processes in Which Noninvasive Ventilation May Be Recommended

Both acute and chronic conditions may be an indication for the use of noninvasive ventilation. From an acute perspective, COPD exacerbation, asthma, and cardiogenic pulmonary edema are disease conditions in which noninvasive ventilation may be used or trialed before escalating to invasive support. Additionally, hypercarbic respiratory failure, post-extubation respiratory failure, and postoperative respiratory failure may all benefit from a closely monitored trial of noninvasive ventilation before considering invasive support. Noninvasive ventilation may also be used in end-of-life care when it is used to minimize respiratory distress and improve patient comfort. For chronic conditions, noninvasive ventilation can be used for COPD, sleep apnea, nocturnal hypoventilation syndrome, and degenerative muscular diseases.

Indications for Changing a Patient to Airway Pressure Release Ventilation

Airway pressure release ventilation is an advanced mode of ventilation that is implemented in patients with severe lung disease or infection, such as Acute Respiratory Distress Syndrome. The goal of Airway Pressure Release Ventilation (APRV) is to increase oxygenation by applying a higher mean airway pressure to the airways without causing increased lung damage by the repeated expansion and relaxation of the lungs with large, vent-controlled breaths. APRV is used in patients with ARDS who fail to improve with conventional ventilation modes. When available, patients are switched to ARPV either in conjunction with or after failure of other interventions, such as increased sedation, prone positioning, or airway clearance therapies. Patients with hemodynamic instability may not tolerate APRV due to the higher intrathoracic pressure and the need for additional vasoactive support.

Narcotic and Benzodiazepine Antagonists

Some drugs such as narcotics and benzodiazepines are associated with serious adverse events including respiratory depression and subsequent death. The abuse and overdose of these medications can result in the need for a reversal agent. Some common narcotic antagonists or reversal agents include naloxone (Narcan) and naltrexone. A common benzodiazepine antagonist or reversal agent is flumazenil. These drugs override and reverse the effects of the narcotic or benzodiazepine, allowing the patient to resume normal breathing and prevent death. It is important to note that although these medications are helpful in reducing drug-related death, they are not always successful.

Utilize Evidence-Based Practice

Mechanical Ventilation Strategies in ARDS Patients Based on the ARDSnet Recommendations

The National Heart, Lung, and Blood Institute has developed recommendations for patients with a diagnosis of Acute Respiratory Distress Syndrome. This collaboration is known as the ARDS network, or ARDSnet. The ARDSnet lists inclusion criteria for their protocol as a P/F ratio of less than or equal to 300, bilateral infiltrates on chest imaging, and no evidence of left atrial hypertension. The first step of the protocol requires calculating a patient's ideal body weight. Tidal volume should initially be adjusted to 8ml/kg and should be weaned down to 6 ml/kg, 1 ml/kg at a time. Respiratory rate should be set to achieve desired minute ventilation, but should not exceed 35 BPM. Tidal volume and respiratory rate should be adjusted to keep the pH greater than 7.15. Goal oxygenation is PaO_2 of 55–80 or SpO_2 of 88–95%. Plateau pressures should remain less than 30 cm H_2O.

Assisting in Preventing Ventilator-Associated Pneumonia

The respiratory therapist has a unique role, as he provides care and interacts with all ventilated patients and is therefore in a position to ensure preventative measures are taken to reduce ventilator-associated pneumonia or ventilator-induced incidents. Proper handwashing and hand hygiene, proper isolation of infectious patients, and surveillance and treatment of infections can decrease cross-contamination between patients. Additionally, the respiratory therapist should ensure the patient's head is elevated 30–45 degrees, keep respiratory equipment clean, provide oral care and secretion removal, and reduce unnecessary disconnection of the ventilator circuit. Closed catheters or inline suction catheters can help maintain clean suction technique and reduce ventilator disconnect frequency. Keeping proper cuff inflation pressures or using the minimum occlusion volume technique with endotracheal tube cuffs can also help minimize drainage of secretions into the lungs.

Alternative Ventilation Strategies for Patients with ARDS

Given the dangers of high respiratory rates and high tidal volumes, permissive hypercapnia can be allowed to prevent long-term lung damage. Inverse I:E ratio is defined by an inspiratory to expiratory ratio usually between 2:1 and 4:1. This allows for recruitment of alveoli and increased mean airway pressure with the goal of improving oxygenation. Airway Pressure Release Ventilation

(APRV) is another method of pressure-controlled ventilation that increases mean airway pressure and oxygenation. This method is preferred over inverse ratio as it is more comfortable for the patient and allows the patient to continue to breathe spontaneously. High-frequency ventilation has had mixed reviews in study outcomes when used in adults with ARDS. However, a tertiary care facility that routinely uses HFV and has more experience with it may have better results. When other methods of mechanical ventilation fail, extracorporeal (ECMO) oxygenation and ventilation may be required.

Pharmacological Interventions in Patients with ARDS

The use of sedation is common practice in the ICU for ARDS patients. Recent recommendations include "holidays" from sedation, where sedation is lightened or paused each day to help reduce the buildup of sedation in a patient's system and to help reduce dependency and tolerance of the medications. In addition, it is recommended to use analgesics and antipsychotic medications instead of benzodiazepines as they are less likely to cause neurocognitive issues. A trial of paralytics can be used for patients who remain asynchronous with the ventilator or in severe distress. Inhaled vasodilators and beta-2 agonists have shown no improvement in ventilator days or mortality. Exogenous surfactant delivery has been attempted, but has only shown to transiently improve oxygenation, and given the high cost of medication, is not recommended for ARDS therapy. Intravenous corticosteroids may be beneficial in the early stages if the underlying cause is pulmonary in nature; however, they cannot be recommended for routine use in all patients due to the high risk of adverse reactions.

Proper Nutrition in Patients with Chronic Lung Disease

Proper nutrition is required for any body system to function as it should. Systems that are already compromised due to illness need proper nutrition to function optimally during the healing process. Patients with respiratory disorders, such as COPD, require additional energy to overcome their increased work of breathing. Malnutrition can cause respiratory muscle fatigue and dysfunction. It increases the risk of respiratory infections due to the inability to effectively remove airway secretions, and it can cause changes in the lung tissue and structure. Patients with COPD are at increased risk for malnutrition due to caloric intake issues such as dyspnea while eating and appetite suppression as a medication side effect. They also have increased difficulty in grocery shopping and food preparation and may suffer from depression, which can lead to poor food choices.

Maintenance Treatment Plan for a Patient with Moderately Persistent Asthma

Asthma patients have their disease diagnosed with a category. This category may change as the disease progresses. Categories are defined based on symptom control with or without medication. Moderately persistent asthma is described as daily symptoms with at least one night time awakening per week, daily use of short-acting beta-2 agonists, some limits in normal activities, and a FEV1 between 60–80% predicted on a pulmonary function test. Patients should have a beta-2 agonist for symptoms available as needed, but should not exceed 3–4 times a day. An inhaled corticosteroid should be administered as prescribed 1–2 times a day. A long-acting bronchodilator may also be administered, especially if nighttime symptoms cause sleep disturbances or symptoms affect activities of daily living.

Recommendations for Discontinuing Mechanical Ventilation

When considering discontinuation of mechanical ventilation, the resolution of the initial cause should be the first indicator. Cardiovascular stability and oxygenation status should be evaluated and optimized prior to extubation. Spontaneous breathing trials will help to decide if the patient can properly ventilate himself post extubation, and ideally the FiO_2 will be set at 50% or less. The patient should be able to control secretions post extubation. Electrolyte levels should be assessed and corrected if necessary. The patient should also be able to prove that he can maintain respiratory status post extubation with an adequate drive to breathe and sufficient respiratory muscle strength. When possible, the patient should be extubated during the day so extubation does not occur during normal sleeping hours, ensuring that fatigue does not contribute to respiratory failure.

Benefits of Respiratory Patient-Driven Protocols

Respiratory patient-driven protocols are developed with the assistance of respiratory care leadership and the respiratory medical director. Once created, a patient-driven protocol allows the respiratory therapist to discontinue or order respiratory therapies as needed based on the patient's current condition. These protocols not only allow for quicker evaluation and implementation of needed respiratory therapies, but also for discontinuation of unneeded or non-indicated therapies. Discontinuation of non-indicated therapies can save the hospital and the patient money, allow for redistribution of needed resources throughout the hospital, and lead to faster hospital discharge as the patient progresses along respiratory pathways. Respiratory patient-driven protocols also allow the respiratory therapist to develop patient care plans and increase his own independence, creating an environment of increased respect and greater job satisfaction.

Classifications for COPD Severity

The Global Initiative for Chronic Obstructive Lung Disease (GOLD) classifies COPD severity in four stages for diagnosis and management of the disease. Stage 1, the initial stage, is considered to be mild disease. On a pulmonary function test, the patient will have greater than 80% of the predicted FEV1. In stage 2, the moderate stage, patients present with 50–80% of their predicted FEV1 on a pulmonary function test. Stage 3 is considered severe and patients present with 30–50% of predicted FEV1 on pulmonary function testing. The final stage, stage 4, is very severe with a FEV1 of less than 30% predicted on testing. It is important to note that the FEV1 values used to diagnose disease stage should be performed when the patient is at baseline health level and not during an acute exacerbation.

Criteria for Asthma Diagnosis

Asthma is defined as airway hyperresponsiveness and a reversible airway obstruction caused by inflammation. The diagnosis of asthma is made by clinical assessment and evaluation with lab and breathing tests. No single test is able to diagnosis asthma, so a combination of assessment and history, including severity and frequency of symptoms, are evaluated. Classic asthma symptoms include shortness of breath, wheezing, chest tightness, and cough. Diagnosis of asthma is not made after a single event, but multiple events. Young children will not usually be diagnosed with reactive airway disease until after the age of two and more than two bronchospasm events. In addition, the type of asthma should be evaluated when making a diagnosis such as allergic asthma, exercise-induced asthma, cough variant asthma, occupational asthma, and nocturnal asthma.

Benefits of Providing Evidence-Based Health Care

Evidence-based medicine is the process of providing health care that has been rigorously reviewed and tested. It allows for a critical analysis of the situation to determine the best possible interventions. It not only promotes the clinician's best judgment, but also the most current literature and management solutions. With healthcare rapidly changing, if providers do not keep up with the current literature and research, they may be unknowingly providing less than the best care and will continue to use outdated methods. Case studies and meta-analysis reports can be used to decide if an intervention would work in the current case. Using evidence-based medicine also encourages development of basic standards of care so physicians and health care providers can easily determine what intervention would be best in a given situation.

Features That Should Appear in All Appropriate Respiratory Protocols

In order for respiratory protocols to work as intended, they need strong management and physician backing. The protocols should state clearly and precisely what they intended to accomplish. An algorithm for the respiratory care practitioner's use should be available and easy to follow. The protocols should include decision points to guide the practitioner through the appropriate course of action for each assessment finding. In addition, there should be points to contact the physician or alert him to changes in the patient's condition. The protocols should also state the point at which therapy is completed or no longer indicated. Respiratory protocols should have an assessment completed every shift with a plan of care in place to dictate care for the next 24 hours.

Provide Respiratory Care in High-Risk Situations

Assessment Steps for a Patient with Suspected Loss or Obstruction of Airway

When a suspected loss of airway has occurred, a colormetric $ETCO_2$ detector or capnography device can be placed on the endotracheal tube to check for return of CO_2 during manual resuscitation. Auscultation of breath sounds should be performed to check for the presence of air movement throughout all lung fields. If breath sounds are louder on one side of the chest, tube displacement into a main stem bronchus or pneumothorax should be considered. A suction catheter can be introduced into the airway to check for blockages. The patient's mouth should be assessed to ensure the patient is not biting the tube and that the tube has not kinked in the mouth or oropharynx. If the patient decompensates or the airway needs to be replaced, the tube should be removed and the patient should be manually ventilated via mask until a new airway can be placed.

Assessment for Effective Chest Compressions

Chest compressions should only be performed by trained personnel who can assess when they are needed and perform them effectively. The best way to assess for the effectiveness of chest compressions is for someone to palpate a pulse during the compressions. If a steady pulse can be felt at the carotid or femoral artery, there is adequate perfusion from the compressions. In addition, capnography can be used when rescue breaths are delivered. If compressions are effective, there should be a return of end tidal CO_2, although the result will not be as high as with spontaneous circulation. The goal should be to keep $EtCO_2$ readings greater than 10 mm Hg. Capnography can also be used to note when a patient returns to spontaneous circulation, as the end tidal CO_2 reading usually has a dramatic spike in value and waveform even during compressions. If the patient has an arterial line placed, the waveform can also be monitored and a goal mean arterial pressure can be determined to ensure adequate perfusion.

Emergency Medications That Can Be Delivered via Endotracheal Route

Epinephrine, lidocaine, and vasopressin can be delivered via the endotracheal route during resuscitation in the absence of intravenous or intraosseous access. These medications should only be used during resuscitation in an attempt to increase the heart rate until venous access can be obtained. Administration of any medication via the endotracheal route has various absorption rates and cannot be guaranteed like medicine delivered via IV or IO. In most cases, the delivered dosage will need to be at least doubled when given via the endotracheal tube instead of IV or IO. Just as when the medication is given via IV or IO, it should be followed by saline to ensure that medication does not adhere to the endotracheal tube.

Cardioversion vs. Defibrillation

Cardioversion attempts to reset the heart into a stable rhythm. It is used with lower dosages than defibrillation. Cardioversion is used on patients who have an abnormal rhythm but are considered stable. Most commonly, it is used on patients with stable ventricular tachycardia. Cardioversion is synchronized, meaning that the patient's rhythm is monitored by the cardioversion machine and the shock is delivered at a specific time during the heart cycle when the R wave is detected. If a patient presents in an abnormal rhythm and no pulse, defibrillation is used, at higher doses than cardioversion. Defibrillation should not be used on a patient who presents with asystole. Defibrillation is not synchronous with the patient's rhythm and the shock will be delivered regardless of any detected rhythm by the machine.

When to Attempt Alternative Airways

Alternative airways should be available anywhere an emergency may happen within the hospital, including in diagnostic areas, on code carts, in the emergency department, and within the intensive care units. After 2–3 unsuccessful intubation attempts, the team should discuss alternative airways. Alternative airways include laryngeal mask airways, king airways, and Combitubes. In addition to using as a backup airway when an endotracheal airway cannot be placed, alternative airways can be placed by additional health care providers not skilled in endotracheal intubation while waiting for additional support. Alternate airways can also be used for short-term ventilation, such as bedside or operating room procedures when endotracheal intubation is not needed. Alternative airways should not be attempted for patients with suspected epiglottitis or other life-threatening upper airway obstructions. Laryngeal mask airway:

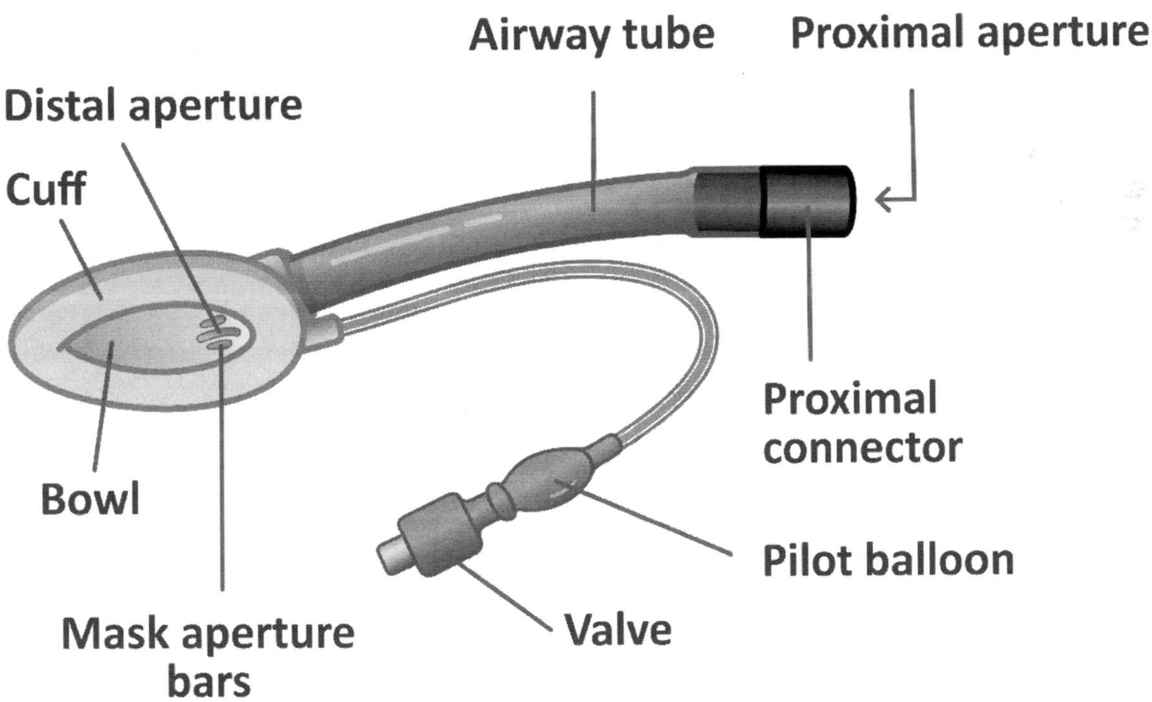

Using Airway Adjuncts in Emergency Situations

Airway adjuncts routinely include oropharyngeal and nasopharyngeal airways. Nasopharyngeal airways are inserted into the nasopharynx to assist with opening the nasal passage and the frequent removal of nasopharyngeal secretions that can occlude the airway. Nasopharyngeal airways can be left in place for hours, or even days, for long-term access to the nasopharynx. Oropharyngeal airways are used to open the mouth and displace the tongue to allow opening of the airway. Oropharyngeal airways can be a great assistance when manual ventilation is needed, but it is important to remember that they should only be used in an unconscious patient as they can induce gagging and vomiting, leading to aspiration. Oropharyngeal airways should only be used short-term until a method for reducing the oral obstruction can be implemented.

Necessary Emergency Equipment When Transporting a Patient with an Artificial Airway Within the Hospital

Any patient with an invasive airway who is being transported through the hospital to a new room, unit, or procedural area should have a respiratory therapist available to make sure the endotracheal tube remains secured and proper oxygenation and ventilation is provided during the transport. Regardless of whether the patient is transported on a ventilator, he should be transported with a manual resuscitator with appropriate size mask in case of emergency. In addition, portable suction, suction catheter, and end tidal CO_2 device should be available in case of questionable tube obstruction or dislodgement. If the destination does not have immediate access to intubation equipment, it should be transported with the patient. The possibility of sedation to keep the patient calm and airway secured should be discussed prior to leaving.

Environmental Factors Affecting the Respiratory System When Transporting a Patient Via Ambulance or Aircraft

Critical care transport of patients from hospital to hospital is used when a higher level of specialized care is needed. In addition to the standard work hazards, providers must be aware of additional factors during transport. Ambulances and aircraft produce strong fumes that can be disrupting to a patient's respiratory status and can induce respiratory distress. Altitude changes can also impact air quality and emergency devices, such as endotracheal tube cuffs and chest tubes. If a patient has a known pneumothorax, it should be decompressed prior to entering an aircraft as high altitudes can make this issue worse. There is also limited working space in transport vehicles, so emergency equipment needs to be easily reached. Providers need to be cognizant of the limited supply of medical air and oxygen on board transport vehicles and to ensure there is ample supply to complete the transport. Finally, all providers should be aware of emergency procedures for both aircraft and ambulance.

Assist a Physician/Provider in Performing Procedures

Equipment to Gather Before Performing/Assisting an Oral Intubation on an Adult Patient

Prior to intubation, all necessary and emergency equipment should be collected, tested, and set up for use at the bedside. Oxygen devices for preoxygenation should be available, including a nasal cannula or non-rebreather mask. A manual resuscitation device should be connected to 100% oxygen for use when the patient has been paralyzed. A laryngoscope blade and handle of appropriate size should be checked and maintained on a clean surface until use. An endotracheal tube of appropriate size, along with one size smaller, should be available with a stylet. Once the endotracheal tube is placed, verification must be performed with a stethoscope and a CO_2 colormetric or capnography device. A way to secure the endotracheal tube should also be available—tape or a commercial tube holder. Both oral and endotracheal suction devices should be available and ready for use. Oral and adjunct airways should be available in case intubation is not possible.

Proper Patient Positioning for Endotracheal Intubation for Patients with/without Suspected Spinal Injury

For a patient without suspected spinal injury, the ideal position for the patient is the sniffing position. A head-tilt/chin-lift can be performed to open the airway and align the upper airway into a more linear position. If the patient is unconscious, an oral airway can be placed to assist while manually ventilating. A towel roll or pillow can be placed under the patient's shoulders to facilitate the correct position. If a spinal injury is suspected, it is important to keep the neck in a neutral position. A jaw thrust can be performed to open the airway and cricoid pressure may be applied to carefully bring the airway into the visual field. A fiberoptic or video intubation device can be used to help with visualization and minimize movement of the patient during the procedure.

Assisting Physicians with a Bronchoscopy

The respiratory therapist plays an important role in assisting the physician in a bronchoscopy. Prior to the procedure, the respiratory therapist should review the order and the patient's medical history, including any contraindications, medications, or disease processes that could cause issues during the procedure. In addition, the therapist should ensure proper functioning of all equipment and emergency supplies. Oxygen and medications should be easily accessible. A "time-out" should be performed to ensure the right patient and the right procedure. During the procedure, the respiratory therapist assists with monitoring the patient's vitals and monitoring for complications. The respiratory therapist also assists with the collection, labeling, and sending of any samples collected. Following the procedure, the therapist should observe for airway compromise, clean and sterilize equipment used, and document the procedure in the patient's medical record.

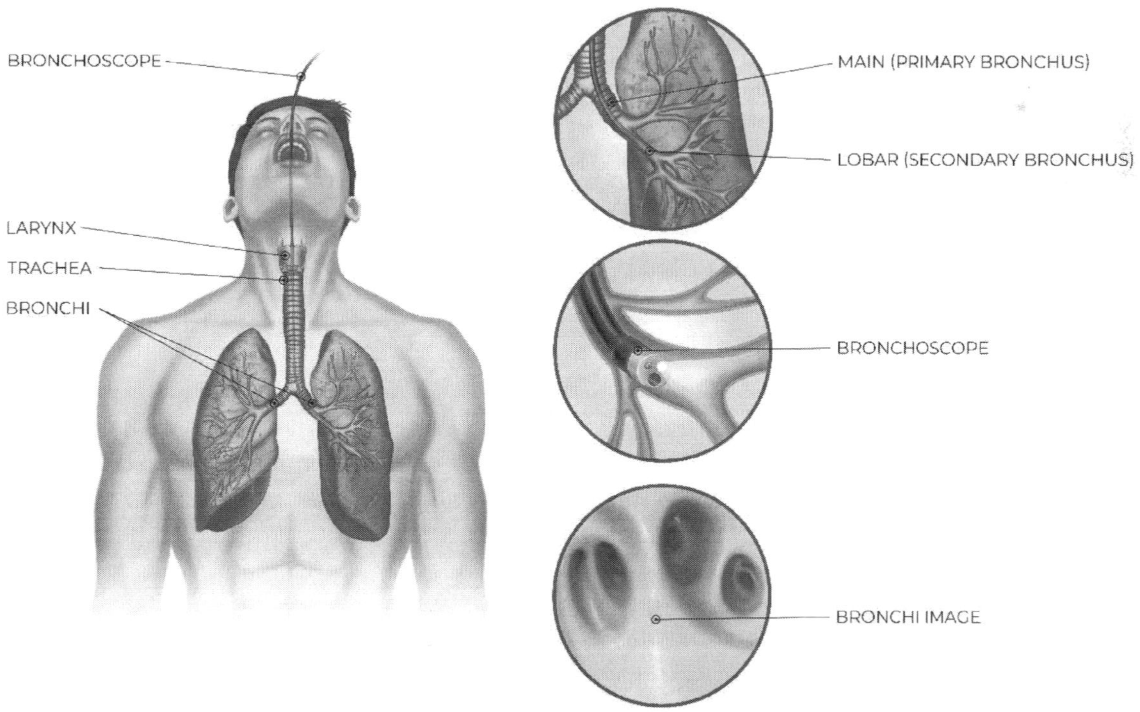

Respiratory Therapist Role When Assisting with Conscious Sedation

Conscious sedation is a frequent procedure in the critical care and emergency department settings. It can be done for setting broken bones or joints, central line placement, endoscopy procedures, and even imaging tests such as MRI's. The respiratory therapist is commonly present to monitor the patient's cardiopulmonary status during the procedure. Oxygen is usually applied as a preventative measure since the respiratory drive may be decreased during the administration of sedation. It is also helpful for the respiratory therapist to use a nasal cannula capnography device to monitor the patient's exhaled carbon dioxide. If the carbon dioxide begins to rise, the physician should be alerted to a decrease in the patient's respiratory drive and the patient may need to be manually ventilated for the remainder of the procedure, or sedation reversal may need to be administered.

Mechanism of Action Behind Cardioversion

Cardioversion is a synchronized electrical shock delivered to the heart when the patient is in an abnormal heart rhythm, unresponsive to medication. Cardioversion synchronizes with the patient's R wave to deliver a shock at precisely the right time. If the shock is delivered during the refractory phase, the patient may convert to ventricular fibrillation or ventricular tachycardia. The rhythms most commonly treated with cardioversion are atrial fibrillation, supraventricular tachycardia, atrial flutter, and monomorphic ventricular tachycardia with a pulse. Cardioversion is indicated when a pulse is present but the patient is starting to shows signs of decrease in consciousness or hypotension or has failed drug therapy. Cardioversion should only be performed by a trained provider in an environment in which further resuscitation can be quickly performed if needed.

Assessments to Be Performed Prior to, During, and after Placing a Patient Prone

Placing a patient prone is used to help increase oxygenation in patients with severe Acute Respiratory Distress Syndrome (ARDS). Placing patients prone can be difficult, given their instability and the number of intravenous lines and ventilator tubing present. Proning a patient takes planning and multiple personnel to minimize the risk to the patient. The patient's vital signs should be continuously monitored to assess tolerance of turning. All lines and tubes on the patient should be monitored to prevent accidental dislodgement. After the patient is placed prone, ventilator graphics and volumes/pressures should be assessed for any changes that may need to be adjusted due to changes in resistance or compliance after changing position. Patients in Pressure Control are especially susceptible to changes in delivered tidal volume, either decreased or increased, following proning.

Indications for Performing a Flexible Bronchoscopy

Flexible bronchoscopes can be fiberoptic, video, or a combination of the two. Flexible bronchoscopy is routinely performed for patients at the bedside in the intensive care units, but can also be used in the outpatient setting with conscious sedation or under general anesthesia. Frequent indications for flexible bronchoscopy include new or unresolving infiltrates on radiographic imaging, diagnosing or staging of cancers, unresolved hemoptysis, airway clearance unresponsive to conventional methods, and evaluation of upper or lower airway abnormalities. Bronchoscopies can be diagnostic or therapeutic. Bronchoalveolar lavage can be performed by instilling a sterile solution into the airways through the flexible bronchoscopy and then aspirating the fluid back. This solution can then be sent to the lab for pathology or culture when a standard sputum sample cannot be obtained through conventional methods.

Proper Positioning of a Patient When Assisting with Portable Chest X-Ray

Positioning of a patient for chest x-ray can have a major effect on the quality of the image and interpretation of line placements. When evaluating the endotracheal tube, the patient's position should be taken into account. If the head and chin are down to the chest, the tip of the endotracheal tube will appear to be lower. If the patient is hyperextended with the chin pointing up, the tip of the tube will appear to be higher than it actually is. To reduce this discrepancy, the patient should be standing or sitting up as much as possible, ideally greater than 45 degrees. All lines and tubes, especially those containing metal pieces, should be lifted off the patient's chest to reduce the possibility of foreign objects appearing on the chest x-ray. The patient should be centered, with hips and clavicles straight. If possible, the x-ray should be taken on full inspiration, and if on the ventilator, an inspiratory hold can be performed if needed.

Assisting Endobronchial Ultrasound and Navigational Bronchoscopy Procedures

An endobronchial ultrasound is a test in which ultrasound waves are applied to the chest during bronchoscopy to help assess the health and structures of the lungs and airways. The use of ultrasound during bronchoscopies is also helpful in navigating a transbronchial needle aspiration because the structures are more clearly visible to clinicians. Similarly, navigational bronchoscopy is a test that helps in visualizing and assessing the smallest airways in the lungs. This specialized test uses a smaller scope than a traditional bronchoscopy procedure, which is able to advance deeper into the lung structures. When assisting during a bronchoscopy, with or without endobronchial ultrasound, the clinician should be prepared to pass the physician tools and saline "bullets," suction the airway as needed, provide supplemental oxygen as needed, and monitor the patient for any changes in oxygen saturation, breathing, alertness, and general comfort.

Conduct Patient and Family Education

Learning Objectives for Asthma Disease Management Education

Asthma education is a key component of disease management to prevent asthma exacerbations and hospitalizations. Asthma education should include the following components: triggers (environmental, seasonal, allergic), signs and symptoms of an asthma attack, peak flow meter use and what the results mean in relation to lung function, names of medication, reasons for and frequency of use, demonstration of proper use of inhalers and nebulizers, importance of cleaning equipment and patient environment, and smoking cessation for patient and family members if needed. Patients should also be able to verbalize the difference between controller medications and rescue medications, when to call physicians, and when to report to an emergency room. Many asthmatics also choose to document times that the rescue inhaler is needed so that symptoms can be tracked and additional long-term medications can be prescribed if needed.

Evaluating Whether the Patient Has Achieved the Learning Objectives

Patient education is important in preventing emergency room visits and hospital readmissions, improving a patient's quality of life, and reducing morbidity and mortality. In addition, quality patient education can lead to lower healthcare costs and medication and therapy compliance. When evaluating a patient's understanding, have the patient explain the disease process in his own words, as well as frequency and purpose of any current medications, signs and symptoms of disease recurrence or episodic flare up, and what to do when these symptom flares happen (emergency room, call to physician, medication). In addition to verbal understanding, the patient should be able to demonstrate proper technique for medication administration and proper disassembly, cleaning, assembly, and application of medical equipment, including oxygen, nebulizers and MDI spacers, CPAP/BiPAP machine, and/or ventilator.

Benefits of Enrolling Patients with Chronic Respiratory Diseases into a Pulmonary Rehabilitation Program

Pulmonary rehabilitation programs combine supervised physical activity with patient education, as well as serving as a support group for those with breathing difficulties. Pulmonary rehabilitation can be beneficial for a wide range of pulmonary issues, including COPD, pulmonary fibrosis, and bronchiectasis. Pulmonary rehabilitation has been shown to increase quality of life, decrease emergency room visits and hospitalization, improve baseline lung function and physical endurance, and improve patients' overall wellbeing and mood. Pulmonary rehabilitation has also been shown to improve outcomes when completed prior to and following an organ transplant, due to the patient's physical improvement. Advances in pulmonary rehabilitation are now expanding into home health services and virtual health services with home-based programs that can reach patients otherwise unable to attend due to transportation or scheduling issues.

Benefits of a Respiratory Therapist in the Home Care Environment

The respiratory therapist can assist patients in their home environment with a better quality of life. Assessment by a trained provider can help patients identify early changes in lung function or sputum production and can help prevent emergency room visits and hospitalizations. For patients receiving respiratory medications, visits from a respiratory therapist can help with compliance of scheduled medications and proper education and administration instructions. For patients requiring advanced technology, such as mechanical ventilation, both invasive and noninvasive, a respiratory therapist can help assure proper functioning of equipment and identify whether to change ventilator settings. Respiratory therapists can also help with equipment inspection, identify potential issues, and get replacement parts before they break and the patient is no longer able to use them. Home pulmonary rehabilitation program follow-ups keep the patient moving and help the benefits of a rehab program last longer.

Importance of Patient Compliance with Sleep Apnea Treatment

Sleep apnea is a serious disease that can be underemphasized by health care providers. Patient compliance with sleep apnea treatment can have a profound impact on quality of life. When sleep apnea treatment is followed, it can lead to more energy and less daytime sleepiness, improved mood, reduction in morning headaches, and better nutritional choices. Untreated sleep apnea can lead to pulmonary hypertension, right heart failure, increased risk of heart attack or stroke, and increased risk of dementia and other cognitive problems. Additionally, patients who fail to follow sleep apnea treatment recommendations have increased morbidity and mortality. When deciding on therapy, it may be necessary to trial multiple patient interface devices to determine which the patient will be most likely to use and stay compliant with.

Influence of a Patient's Culture on Education and Healthcare

A patient's culture has an impact on behaviors that can affect health and wellbeing. Beliefs that can impact health include causes of disease or illness (negative thoughts, imbalances in life forces, curses, etc.), social impacts (gay, bisexual, transgender), family (fear of disownment or going against family wishes), and treatment options (refusal of blood products, organ retrieval, or organ donation). In addition, it may be necessary to consider preference for same sex providers, only male physicians, or presence of religious clergy. Culture may also affect the language and health literacy skills of the patient. Documentation of care discussions should be done in a language the patient is comfortable with. Finally, body language varies tremendously among different cultures and should be taken into account when deciding if the patient has understood the education. The appropriateness of eye contact, body closeness, and asking questions can vary between cultures.

Exercise and the Treatment of Respiratory Diseases

Exercise is an important component of a healthy lifestyle, especially for patients with respiratory diseases. Being overweight or obese can contribute to poorly controlled asthma and chronic obstructive pulmonary disease. Excess weight, especially around the chest and abdomen, can cause a restrictive effect, reducing a patient's lung capacity. Excess weight also contributes to gastroesophageal reflux disease, which is a severe form of acid reflux. This reflux causes inflammation in the lungs, resulting in more severe and poorly controlled asthma symptoms. Exercise should be promoted by the clinical staff, but it should be started gradually so that a patient does not suffer from exercise-induced bronchospasm or overexertion and subsequent severe shortness of breath.

Cystic Fibrosis

Cystic fibrosis, a hereditary respiratory disease associated with excess secretions and increased levels of immunoreactive trypsinogen, is a lifelong disorder that sometimes requires a lung transplant. Patients with cystic fibrosis often have a reduced lifespan; however, current medical guidelines have helped prolong these patients' lives with proper treatment. Treatment for cystic fibrosis includes chest physiotherapy, often via "vest" technology, bronchodilators, enzyme supplements, antimicrobial nebulizer treatments during exacerbations, and inhaled steroids. Symptom severity and infection frequency vary widely among patients with cystic fibrosis, and there is no one-size-fits-all therapy. However, most patients use a combination of the aforementioned therapies to keep their symptoms under control and prevent exacerbations. Patients with cystic fibrosis are often hospitalized during infections, and they may be in isolation due to the presence of *Pseudomonas aeruginosa*, which is a common infection associated with cystic fibrosis.

Ventilator-Dependent Patients

Patients who are ventilator dependent are found in facilities such as nursing homes and hospitals, but they may also be treated at home or in hospice care. Clinicians should be aware of the special challenges associated with these patients so that they are treated effectively and appropriately. Ventilator checks may be performed by respiratory therapists. Clinicians should ensure that the ventilator settings are appropriate and have remained unchanged since the last check. Clinicians must evaluate the patient with a full physical assessment to determine any change from the last visit. This can include changes in oxygenation that may require oxygen titration, changes in breath sounds that may require treatment with bronchodilators, and signs of infection. The airway must stay patent, and it may require tracheostomy care if a tracheostomy tube is in use. Otherwise, the patient will require suctioning of the endotracheal tube. Mechanical ventilation can also be provided noninvasively via a mask. These patients often use the ventilator only at night for the treatment of central sleep apnea.

Challenges Associated with the Treatment of Patients with Lung Cancer

The severity of symptoms of patients with lung cancer varies widely depending on the stage of the cancer and on patients' overall health. Severe symptoms and more advanced lung cancer stages can result in a patient being placed in hospice or other inpatient care facilities. Treatment for lung cancer is also dependent on the stage of the cancer, but it can include interventions such as lumpectomy and other surgical procedures, chemotherapy, and radiation. Patients with lung cancer may require supplemental oxygen in the home or clinical setting due to hypoxemia secondary to the disease. Some patients may also benefit from bronchodilator therapy, which helps to dilate the airways and reduce shortness of breath.

CRT/RRT Practice Test

1. Upon review of the patient record, the respiratory therapist notices that the chart indicates that the patient has a code status of "Do not resuscitate." During a routine assessment, the patient becomes apneic, and subsequently asystolic. Which of these should the respiratory therapist do?

a. Begin bag-mask ventilation with an FiO_2 of 1.00 and a flow of 15 L/min.
b. Call for emergency intubation, and initiate mechanical ventilation.
c. Begin chest compressions.
d. Report this to the charge nurse as soon as possible.

2. A review of physician orders for a patient admitted to an acute care facility with an exacerbation of chronic obstructive pulmonary disease (COPD) shows that the medications ordered include Combivent q4h and DuoNeb q4h. The respiratory therapist has a responsibility to perform which of these actions?

a. Dispense/administer medication as ordered.
b. Contact the ordering physician to verify orders.
c. Alternate medications every two hours.
d. Do not administer whichever medication is contraindicated.

3. Upon having difficulty getting a reading with the finger probe of a pulse oximeter, the respiratory therapist decides to check the patient's peripheral circulation and capillary refill. The nail bed on the right index finger, after a brief compression, becomes pink again after one second. This is an indication of which of the following?

a. insufficient blood flow to extremities
b. normal peripheral circulation and capillary refill
c. anemia
d. cyanosis

4. A 20-year-old female patient is brought to the emergency department (ED) by paramedics after suffering a brief loss of consciousness after a collision with another player on the basketball court. Upon arrival, the patient's SpO_2 is 98% on room air, her respiratory rate is 16, and her heart rate is 95. The venous blood draw shows that hemoglobin is 11.0 and hematocrit is 44. How do you report these findings?

a. Patient is saturating well on room air and has a normal heart rate and respiratory rate. Hemoglobin and hematocrit are within normal limits.
b. Patient is saturating well on room air and has a normal heart rate and respiratory rate. Hemoglobin is low at 11.0, and hematocrit is within normal limits.
c. Patient is saturating well on room air and is tachypneic with a normal heart rate. Hemoglobin and hematocrit are within normal limits.
d. Patient is saturating well on room air and is tachycardic at 95 with a normal respiratory rate. Hemoglobin is high at 11.0, and hematocrit is within normal limits.

5. The first patient we see today for an evaluation is a 45-year-old female who started smoking cigarettes at age 15. She reports that she smokes one and a half packs a day and that she quit for a year when she was pregnant with each or her two children. Her husband is also a smoker. How do you report this smoking history in the patient chart?

a. Patient is currently a daily cigarette smoker, 1.5 packs per day, with a 42-pack-year history.
b. Patient is currently a heavy smoker.
c. Patient smokes about 30 cigarettes a day and has for almost 30 years.
d. Patient suffers from a nicotine addiction and smokes too much.

6. When introducing herself to a patient for the first time, the respiratory therapist notices that the patient is only able to respond to questions in two- or three-word phrases, breaking up longer responses to take breaths after every couple of words. What conclusions can the respiratory therapist safely make from this speech pattern?

a. The patient is most likely not a native English speaker
b. The patient has a decreased vital capacity, and there could be several different causes for this.
c. The patient has COPD.
d. The patient has a neuromuscular illness that impairs respiration.

7. Auscultation of breath sounds during an examination of a 20-year-old male reveals high-pitched wheezing throughout the lung field. The patient reports that he is slightly short of breath and that the wheezing, though noticeable, bothers him very little. He notices that it usually happens when he mows the lawn. Which of the following might we recommend to the physician?

a. Write a prescription for an albuterol inhaler to use when necessary (pro re nata [PRN]).
b. Send the patient for a chest X-ray (CXR) and full pulmonary function tests (PFTs).
c. The best course is to "wait and see" for this minor problem.
d. The patient's respiratory health is uncertain and would be better understood by performing basic spirometry and a methacholine challenge test.

8. A 50-year-old female patient presents with a three-month history of a cough productive of sputum that is more acute in the morning upon waking. The sputum is moderate in consistency, pale yellow in color, and varies from small to moderate in quantity. There is no fever or recent sick contacts. Auscultation reveals scattered rhonchi bilaterally, mostly in the lower lobes. The patient has no smoking history. What do you recommend?

a. A more complete history including vocation, exposure to environmental hazards, and family history is required. Also, PFTs are indicated for this patient with a pre- and post-bronchodilator FEV1/FVC.
b. Tell the physician that the patient has COPD and needs a long-acting beta agonist and an inhaled corticosteroid to start at once.
c. An order for a stat CXR and a complete blood count (CBC) with differential is necessary to rule out pneumonia.
d. The patient needs pulmonary rehabilitation with exercise and nutritional counseling.

9. A patient presents to the ED of your hospital with productive cough, fever, and bilateral rhonchi in the lower lobes. The CXR shows possible bilateral infiltrate, according to the radiologist. To confirm a diagnosis of pneumonia, what level of white blood cells (WBCs) would we expect to find per microliter (mcL)?

a. 2,000 to 3,000 WBCs/mcL
b. 4,000 to 6,000 WBCs/mcL
c. 7,000 to 10,000 WBCs/mcL
d. 12,000 to 14,000 WBCs/mcL

10. While performing routine care on a patient with a tracheostomy, you notice that there are traces of blood apparent on the dressing between the stoma and the flange of the tube. Which of these is the correct course of action?

a. Put on a new, clean dressing and set a reminder to check for additional problems when doing tracheostomy care the following day.
b. Clean the area of the stoma with normal saline; do a careful inspection of the condition of the stoma; replace the old dressing with a new, clean dressing; carefully note your observation in the patient chart; and directly notify the unit manager that the stoma needs the attention of the patient's physician or advanced practice registered nurse (APRN) when one of them next does rounds.
c. Clean the area of the stoma with a cotton swab saturated with hydrogen peroxide and sterile water in a 50/50 mix; replace the dressing with a clean, new dressing; and ask that the patient be seen by the physician on call stat.
d. Continue regular tracheostomy care as per usual protocol, make a mental note of the trace blood, and tell the next therapist about it when you give your report at the change of shift.

11. A patient brought into the ED by paramedics from a car accident appears to have possibly suffered a chest wall injury. The physician orders an arterial blood gas (ABG) analysis (on room air). The results come back as follows:

pH	7.24
$PaCO_2$	58 mm Hg
PaO_2	84 mm Hg
HCO_{3-}	24 mEq/L

What respiratory treatment might we recommend to the physician?

a. Stat CXR and possible noninvasive positive pressure ventilation (NIPPV)
b. Supplemental O_2 at 5 L/min via nasal cannula
c. Stat intubation and mechanical ventilation
d. CXR and 2 L/min supplemental O_2 via nasal cannula

12. A patient in your care has appropriate tidal volumes; clear bilateral breath sounds throughout his lung fields; normal CBC; no signs or symptoms of infection; and although he is on a venturi mask delivering an FiO_2 of 0.45, he has an SpO_2 of 87%. The patient chart shows a history of a clotting disorder, although he is not currently taking an anticoagulant. What test would you recommend be performed next?

a. prothrombin time (PT) and international normalized ratio (INR)
b. ventilation-perfusion (V/Q) scan
c. CXR
d. ultrasound exam of aorta and echocardiogram

13. A patient in the telemetry unit sets off an alarm when her SpO_2 drops below 90% — all the way to 85%. The patient has a No. 6 Shiley tracheostomy tube in place; she has a disposable inner cannula in place, and the cuff is deflated. Upon entering her room, what is the first thing you must do?

a. Assess the patient for signs of distress and check the pulse oximetry probe to see that it is securely in place.
b. Check that the FiO_2 setting on the entrainment device is set properly, as ordered.
c. Begin bag-mask ventilation with 100% oxygen at 15 L/min.
d. Attempt to pass a suction catheter through the tracheostomy tube to remove accumulated secretions and to ensure that the tube is patent.

14. Acute on chronic lung disease is best shown in which of the following arterial blood gas (ABG) results (on 4 L/min O_2 via nasal cannula)?

a.	pH 7.36	PO_2 86	PCO_2 52	HCO_3 30
b.	pH 7.11	PO_2 79	PCO_2 61	HCO_3 24
c.	pH 7.40	PO_2 70	PCO_2 40	HCO_3 25
d.	pH 7.30	PO_2 91	PCO_2 52	HCO_3 26

15. If we need to determine a patient's functional residual capacity (FRC), which of these tests should the physician order?

a. bedside spirometry
b. ABG analysis
c. V/Q scan
d. body plethysmography

16. A patient is sent for pulmonary function testing to confirm or refute a tentative diagnosis of COPD. The test is ordered to be performed pre- and post-bronchodilator. What minimum degree of change in forced vital capacity (FVC) do we need to see in order to conclude that there is a significant difference attributable to the bronchodilator?

a. 4%
b. 8%
c. 10%
d. 12%

17. When calibrating the spirometer in the pulmonary function laboratory, the respiratory therapist performs three trials with a 3 L syringe. The results are 2.92 L, 3.02 L, and 3.09 L. What does the respiratory therapist report about the spirometer as a result of these measurements?

a. It needs service and should not be used.
b. It is in good working order.
c. It is working erratically and needs to be checked by the supervisor.
d. Using the device is not safe at this time.

18. Mrs. Galvez is a 70-year-old Hispanic woman with a 50-pack-year smoking history. Her physician has sent her to you with an order for full pulmonary function testing because she presented to him with a persistent, productive cough. Her FVC is within normal range for her height/age/race. Her FEV_1/FVC is 0.61, or 61% of normal. What does this number suggest?

a. Mrs. Galvez should be sent for a stat CXR.
b. The patient's effort was inadequate.
c. Mrs. Galvez has a sign of an obstructive lung disorder, possibly severe COPD.
d. Mrs. Galvez has a sign of an obstructive lung disorder, possibly moderate COPD.

19. A patient is brought into the ED by paramedics after a one-car motor vehicle accident. The patient was the driver. He is a 20-year-old male, conscious but lethargic. He is complaining of severe pain in his right leg, neck, and chest. The stat CXR shows tracheal deviation to the right side. What is a possible cause of the X-ray findings?

a. elevated hemidiaphragm
b. right middle lobe atelectasis
c. right-side pneumothorax
d. left-side pneumothorax

20. A 35-year-old female patient is brought into the ED by her family. They suspect she may have taken an overdose of heroin. The physician wants to check for possible hypoventilation as a result of a suppressed respiratory drive and orders an ABG. In what order do we perform these steps?

a. Check for written order, check patient ID, prepare ABG draw kit, perform Allen's test, wash hands, glove, clean site with alcohol swab, draw sample.
b. Perform Allen's test, check for written order, check patient ID, prepare ABG draw kit, wash hands, glove, clean puncture site with alcohol swab, draw sample.
c. Check for written order, check patient ID, wash hands, perform Allen's test, wash hands again, glove, prepare ABG draw kit, clean site with alcohol swab, draw sample.
d. Check patient ID, perform Allen's test, check for written order, wash hands, glove, prepare ABG draw kit, clean site with alcohol swab, draw sample.

21. Which of the following conditions in a patient chart might cause you to suspect that a high SPO_2 reading from a pulse oximeter might not be accurate for a particular patient?

a. The patient is a smoker who stepped out for a cigarette immediately before the examination.
b. The patient works as a firefighter.
c. The patient's hemoglobin on a recent CBC was 14.9.
d. The patient is wearing dark nail polish.

22. The pulmonologist has ordered bedside spirometry for a patient on his service. The patient is a 29-year-old male smoker admitted through the ED after a diagnosis was made of ethanol toxicity. The patient is 183 cm tall, Caucasian, and weighs 105 kg. Three trials yield the following results for FVC and FEV_1:

4.70 L/4.00 L	5.67 L/4.66 L	4.01 L/3.96 L

The Centers for Disease Control and Prevention's Third National Health and Nutrition Examination Survey (NHANES III) predicted value is 5.84 L/4.75 L. What should the respiratory therapist report to the physician?

a. Inconsistent patient effort precludes useful analysis.
b. The spirometry is normal for the age/height/race.
c. Obstructive disease is evident.
d. Restrictive disease is evident.

23. Your patient is an 18-year-old recent immigrant from the Philippines. Due to findings on the patient's CXR and the symptoms he presented with upon initial examination, the physician has given the patient a tentative diagnosis of tuberculosis and has admitted the patient to the hospital, ordering additional tests and appropriate isolation precautions. Which personal protective equipment (PPE) must we use during contact with this patient?

a. N-95 mask, gown, gloves
b. surgical mask, gown, gloves
c. gown, gloves
d. N-95 mask, gown, gloves, bonnet, booties

24. A 14-year-old African-American female with a diagnosis of asthma has, with your guidance and assistance, prepared an asthma action plan. Her daily peak flow measurements are recorded each morning. What results would indicate she is in the "yellow zone" and needs to use her inhaler according to the plan?

a. a peak flow reading 15% lower than her best
b. a peak flow reading 25% lower than her best
c. a peak flow reading 55% lower than her best
d. an inability to perform a peak flow maneuver

25. Pulmonary function testing should be postponed for all of the following patients except:

a. 71-year-old male, status/post cerebrovascular accident (CVA) one week
b. 17-year-old female, recent CXR showing right-sided pneumothorax
c. 33-year-old female, two broken ribs from a fall three days ago
d. 15-year-old male, recent respiratory infection

26. During the analysis of the flow-volume curve of a patient's pulmonary function testing, we suspect that the patient may have coughed during the first second of exhale during one of the trials. What indicator would we see in the graph to lead to this conclusion?

a. a jagged interruption or dip in the curve during exhale
b. a steep slope of the line during the expiratory phase of the maneuver
c. an unusually high value for FVC1
d. a diminished value for FVC1

27. The physician has asked us to evaluate the respiratory status of a patient with muscular dystrophy. Of all the tests that we may use in this assessment, which one should be performed first?

a. maximum inspiratory pressure (MIP)
b. maximal voluntary ventilation (MVV)
c. arterial blood gas (ABG)
d. CXR

28. When examining the flow-time graph of Mr. LaGuardia's pulmonary function test, we see that the line noticeably declines toward the baseline after reaching a plateau. What does this indicate?

a. poor patient effort
b. blockage in the mouthpiece
c. a likely leak in the circuit
d. obstructive lung disorder

29. The physician has asked for assistance in diagnosing a patient with moderate respiratory distress, a productive cough, and a fever. The patient coughs and expectorates sputum, which should always be examined for which characteristics?

a. color
b. odor
c. consistency
d. culture

30. When ABG results reveal that the patient is alkalotic, although she is apparently breathing normally, a possible cause is

a. repeated vomiting
b. hypoventilation
c. blood loss
d. internal bleeding

31. A patient in the telemetry unit is on continuous monitoring for, among other vital signs, SpO_2. The patient has no signs of hypoxemia or respiratory distress but is now setting off an alarm when the SpO_2 reading dips to 80% on 28% O_2 via nasal cannula. A stat ABG shows a PaO_2 of 85 mmHg. What course of action is indicated?

a. Increase FiO_2.
b. Decrease FiO_2.
c. Disregard the pulse-oximeter reading and maintain the same FiO_2.
d. Repeat the ABG.

32. You want to assess the ventilatory status of a long-term mechanical ventilator patient in a skilled nursing facility. An ABG analysis is not available in house and would require the patient be sent to a pulmonary laboratory. The next best choice would be which of these tests?

a. end-tidal CO_2 levels measured with capnography
b. finger probe pulse oximetry
c. HCO_3 and CO_2 levels in a venous blood draw
d. examination of patient for central or peripheral cyanosis

33. A full polysomnography study in a properly equipped sleep lab will include continuous monitoring and recording of which of these sets of parameters?

a. respiratory rate, heart rate, blood pressure, blood glucose
b. heart rate, leg movement, snoring, SpO_2, chest expansion
c. brain activity, air flow, sleeping position, galvanic skin response
d. end-tidal CO_2, rapid eye movement, airway resistance, vocalizations during sleep

34. The interpretation of the sleep study shows definitive evidence of obstructive sleep apnea. The diagnosis will be made for moderate sleep apnea if the apnea hypopnea index (AHI) is

a. > 5
b. > 10 and < 15
c. > 15 and < 30
d. > 20 and < 45

35. The ICU team is considering whether a metabolic study with indirect calorimetry is indicated for Mr. Pulaski. Which of the following is not included in the patient groups for whom this test may be indicated?

a. patients at the extremes of weight
b. patients with high levels of stress
c. patients who are difficult to wean from the ventilator
d. patients who are typically physically active

36. Which of these vital signs are NOT included in the computation of an Apgar score?

a. muscle tone
b. reflex irritability
c. heart rate
d. pupillary reaction

37. With regard to an assessment of gestational age, the different between a very low birth weight infant (VLBW) and an extremely low birth weight infant (ELBW) is

a. the difference between birthweight < 2,000 g and birthweight < 1,500 g
b. the difference between birthweight < 1,500 g and birthweight < 1,000 g
c. the difference between birthweight < 2,500 g and birthweight < 2,000 g
d. the difference between birthweight < 2,750 g and birthweight < 1,800 g

38. For Ms. Goldberg, whose blood pressure is low and whose cardiac output is decreased, the therapy that is considered before others is

a. IV fluid administration
b. vasopressors
c. inotropic agents
d. diuretics

39. Mr. Esposito has a diagnosis of congestive heart failure, and he is currently experiencing an exacerbation of this condition. How is this likely to be manifested in his respiratory status?

a. He may be difficult to oxygenate due to fluid buildup in his lungs (pulmonary edema).
b. On inspiration, the respiratory therapist will auscultate coarse rhonchi.
c. His airway resistance will increase due to bronchospasm.
d. It will have no effect.

40. When examining the patient for signs of increased work of breathing (WOB), the respiratory therapist must look for all of the following signs or diagnoses except:

a. increased respiratory rate
b. accessory muscle use
c. diagnosis with idiopathic pulmonary fibrosis (IPF)
d. decreased GI function

41. Mrs. Jackson is in the intensive care unit (ICU), and her intracranial pressure (ICP) is being monitored out of concern that it may rise to an unsafe level. Monitoring is accomplished with a miniature pressure transducer inserted in the lateral ventricle. The pressure is dangerously high. We can see her ICP return to a safe baseline level when it decreases from

a. 35 mmHg to 30 mmHg
b. 30 mmHg to 20 mmHg
c. 20 mmHg to 10 mmHg
d. 10 mmHg to 5 mmHg

42. Monitoring an 80-year-old male in the telemetry unit, the respiratory therapist notices on the electrocardiogram (ECG) monitor that the patient's PR interval has increased to 0.22 seconds with an otherwise regular rhythm. A possible cause for this is

a. hypertension
b. dehydration
c. internal bleeding
d. sinus tachycardia

43. When monitoring hemodynamic parameters with a pulmonary artery catheter, which of these values would NOT give us cause for alarm?

a. mean pulmonary artery pressure of 8 mmHg
b. pulmonary capillary wedge pressure of 5 mmHg
c. central venous pressure of 18 mmHg
d. cardiac output of 2 L/min

44. When giving a report on the status of a patient in the ED, the respiratory therapist describes the patient as "A & O x3." This means that during assessment the patient is

a. awake and obtunded
b. aware of time, place and pain
c. alert and oriented to time, place, person
d. alert and oriented to pain, pressure, recent events

45. When asked to describe the pain he is feeling, Mr. Faucher responds, "I have no words to describe what I am feeling." How do we help Mr. Faucher and get a useful assessment of the level of his pain?

a. Ask him if he thinks that it feels like the time he broke a bone.
b. Observe Mr. Faucher for wincing, breath holding, and bulging veins.
c. Check heart rate and blood pressure.
d. Ask the patient to rate his pain on a scale from 1 (very little) to 10 (the worst he's ever had).

46. While we are assessing Mr. Salaam, he tells us he has a cough in the morning, productive of sputum. We ask him what color, and he responds, "I never looked." Why is it important for us to know this to better help our patient?

a. We'll know much he smokes.
b. To see if he's being truthful.
c. The color can be a telltale sign of respiratory infection.
d. If there's no blood in his sputum, he's OK.

47. Mr. Jackson reports an occasional feeling of tightness in his chest that is accompanied by wheezing. He tells us he has never had asthma and that because he is adopted, he doesn't know about a family history of respiratory issues. He has never smoked and lives with a nonsmoking partner. What else must the respiratory therapist ask Mr. Jackson to better help the physician with a diagnosis?

a. What is your work environment like?
b. Are you frequently tense and nervous?
c. Do you consume alcohol every day?
d. Did you receive the pertussis vaccine as a child?

48. Mrs. Hunter tells the respiratory therapist that she spends her day on the sofa watching television. When doing so, she feels no shortness of breath. How do we determine and report her ability to perform activities of daily living (ADLs) with regard to dyspnea?

a. She reports no dyspnea so is not limited by it.
b. She is sedentary and therefore incapable of performing ADLs.
c. We ask her questions about toileting, meal preparation, and simple housework.
d. We call her daughter or son to obtain more objective information.

49. During an evaluation of a 37-year-old female patient who presents with a cough of unknown etiology, which family and personal history question is most relevant?

a. Do you drink?
b. Do you have family history of renal failure?
c. Do you live with smokers?
d. Do you have any food allergies?

50. Tracheal deviation from midline will occur with which of these pairs of disorders?

a. pneumothorax and hemothorax
b. lung cancer and Guillain-Barré syndrome
c. pulmonary edema and atelectasis
d. aspiration of foreign body and pericardial effusions

51. Lateral neck radiographs can assist with the diagnosis of which acute condition?

a. bronchiolitis
b. respiratory syncytial virus
c. croup
d. pertussis

52. Proper patient positioning in a CXR will yield an image that includes all of the following except:

a. Lung apices
b. Costophrenic angles
c. Hemidiaphragms
d. Hyoid

53. The presence of pleural effusions will be seen in the CXR as

a. a light area at the lung base, at the costophrenic angle
b. a dark area at the lung base, at the costophrenic angle
c. ground glass opacity
d. Kerley B lines

54. The difference between an anterior/posterior (A/P) CXR and a posterior/anterior (P/A) CXR is

a. The heart is shown on the opposite side.
b. In an A/P CXR, the heart appears larger.
c. In a P/A CXR, the heart appears larger.
d. The A/P technique distorts the spinal column.

55. A portable CXR shows an elevated hemidiaphragm on the right side. The most common reason this is seen is

a. enlarged liver resulting from cirrhosis
b. gastroenteritis
c. small-bowel obstruction
d. excessive gas accumulated in the stomach

56. The 12-lead ECG is widely used because

a. It is noninvasive and painless.
b. Medicare rules require that each patient receives one.
c. The tracing can tell what the heart is going to do next.
d. They have fewer artifacts than 3- or 5-lead ECGs.

57. A respiratory therapist can determine minute ventilation by first measuring

a. tidal volume and respiratory rate
b. forced expiratory volume and residual volume
c. SpO_2 and respiratory rate
d. inspiratory force and expiratory force

58. A respiratory therapist is assigned to a patient in the ICU who is on continuous mechanical ventilation. Among other parameters charted every two hours is the patient's plateau pressure. Why is this of such great importance for the treatment of this patient?

a. Limiting the plateau pressure reduces the likelihood of lung injury.
b. Maintaining a higher plateau pressure improves oxygenation.
c. A plateau pressure of > 30 cm H_2O is associated with better outcomes.
d. Maintaining a higher P_{PLAT} is associated with fewer instances of lung injury.

59. The alveolar-arterial oxygen tension difference — $(P_A\text{-}P_a)O_2$ — is a measure of gas exchange that is a useful indicator in helping to determine our patient's pulmonary status. In order for us to assess this difference, the respiratory therapist needs to know:

a. DLCO and SpO_2
b. FiO_2 and VT
c. peak pressure and FiO_2
d. PaO_2 and FiO_2

60. Mrs. Papadopoulos has been referred to the cardiac rehabilitation program for cardiopulmonary exercise evaluation (CPX). The respiratory therapist at the program must be aware of the relative contraindications of CPX, which include all of the following except:

a. angina with exercise
b. inability or unwillingness of the patient to participate
c. uncontrolled diabetes
d. mildly elevated BMI

61. On the order of the intensivist on duty in the ICU, a respiratory therapist draws an ABG sample for analysis to see if our patient's minute ventilation is sufficient for maintaining the appropriate PaCO2.

There are numerous errors an inexperienced or poorly trained respiratory therapist might make that would degrade the accuracy or reliability of the analysis; they include which of the following?

a. Waiting more than 20 minutes to analyze the sample
b. Expelling air bubbles from the syringe after the draw
c. Failure to aspirate the sample
d. Noting oxygen delivery system and flow rate, if present

62. During regularly scheduled ventilator checks, the thorough and conscientious respiratory therapist will check the cuff pressure on the endotracheal tube to see that it is neither too high nor too low. The device used to make this measurement is a

a. a built-in feature of the ventilator
b. 10 cc syringe
c. stethoscope for auscultation of the neck/chest
d. manometer

63. Mr. Chao has a suspected respiratory infection that is proving very difficult to precisely diagnose. His physician wants to perform a sputum culture, but the amount of sputum Mr. Chao is able to expectorate is scant or none. What can the respiratory therapist suggest as a method to help obtain a suitable sputum sample?

a. Administer IV hydration to the patient.
b. Administer hypertonic saline (3%) to the patient via nebulizer.
c. Encourage the patient to drink more fluids.
d. Treat the patient with nebulized albuterol (2.5 mg/3 mL H_2O) to dilate the airways.

64. Which one of the following statements is NOT true of patients who are demonstrating auto positive end-expiratory pressure (auto-PEEP) while on mechanical ventilation?

a. The patient most likely has an obstructive lung disorder.
b. The expiratory time is probably too short.
c. Reducing minute ventilation may eliminate the auto-PEEP.
d. Diuresing the patient will reduce the auto-PEEP.

65. According to the American Association for Respiratory Care's clinical practice guidelines, when charting the measurements taken via transcutaneous monitoring of $PtcO_2$ and $PtcCO_2$, it is required that the respiratory therapist chart all of the following except:

a. a subjective assessment of the clinical appearance of the patient
b. the mode of ventilatory support and the settings
c. the FiO_2 (or O_2 flow rate) and the method of oxygen delivery
d. Atmospheric conditions outside

66. The value of performing an overnight pulse oximetry test is demonstrated by its ability to help us determine

a. which patients may have sleep-disordered breathing versus simple snoring
b. which respiratory muscles are not functioning while the patient sleeps
c. the cause of nocturnal O_2 desaturation
d. if the Epworth Sleepiness Scale was properly administered

67. A patient whose respiratory status we are assessing in the ICU is unconscious and unable to cooperate with our efforts. Nevertheless, we can perform which of the following measurements?

a. vital capacity
b. maximum inspiratory pressure
c. FEV1
d. peak expiratory flow

68. Acceptable methods of determining the correct continuous positive airway pressure (CPAP) pressure setting for patients with obstructive sleep apnea include the following:

a. titration in a sleep lab OR titration with an auto-CPAP machine at home
b. titration in a sleep lab ONLY
c. titration with auto-CPAP at home ONLY
d. experimentation with various CPAP settings at home OR titration in a sleep lab

69. A respiratory therapist is evaluating the results of hemoximetry just performed on a patient in the labor and delivery unit. Possible causes of measurement errors that must be considered in the evaluation include all of the following except:

a. sickle cell anemia
b. dirty cuvette chamber
c. high lipid levels from parenteral nutrition
d. hypertension

70. A respiratory therapist has returned to his job at a New England hospital center from a charitable medical mission to Central Africa. A month later, he is experiencing a persistent bad cough with hemoptysis. Which of these tests are likely to be ordered to help diagnose the problem?

a. magnetic resonance imaging (MRI)
b. methacholine provocation
c. purified protein derivative (PPD) test
d. polysomnography

71. A respiratory therapist goes to the supply room to get a nasal cannula for a patient in their care. The liter flow ordered by the physician is 2 L/min. The therapist notes that the expiration date on the packaging of the item shows that it expired just within the last month. The proper immediate course of action for the therapist is

a. Discard the expired nasal cannula, and advise the central supply manager of outdated equipment on the shelves. Then, obtain a nasal cannula that has not reached its stated expiration to supply to this patient.
b. Open the package and assess the condition of the nasal cannula. If all is good upon close examination, use it for the supplemental O_2 for this patient.
c. Discard the nasal cannula, and if there are more than two outdated nasal cannulas on the shelf, notify the state department of health.
d. Ignore the expiration date because a nasal cannula has no moving parts.

72. When setting up a CPAP machine for Mrs. Rose, a new admission, the respiratory therapist is required to inspect the machine for safety, good overall condition, and proper operation. The respiratory therapist notices that although everything appears fine, there is no preventive maintenance (PM) sticker on the CPAP machine. This sticker shows that it was inspected and when it next needs inspection and bench testing by the biomedical department. What action is indicated by the lack of this sticker?

a. Continue setting up the machine for this patient, and then get the biomedical department on the phone to request a sticker
b. Discard the machine and get another one with a current sticker for the use of this patient.
c. Obtain another CPAP machine that has the correct PM sticker, and then see to it that the first one is brought to the attention of the biomedical technicians. Set the machine aside until it can be serviced.
d. Finish setting up the machine, fit the mask to the patient, turn it on, and ask the patient if it feels like the one she has at home.

73. When setting up an ICU room for a new mechanical ventilator patient, the presence of which item is required?

a. incentive spirometer
b. nonrebreather mask
c. bag-mask ventilation device
d. breath-actuated nebulizer

74. A patient on mechanical ventilation in the ICU for the past 24 hours, who is recovering from severe pneumonia, is doing well and her condition seems to be improving each shift. Suddenly and without warning, the high-pressure and low-volume alarms are sounding. One possible cause could be

a. excessive sedation
b. patient biting on the endotracheal (ET) tube
c. decreased airway resistance
d. a sudden drop in the plateau pressure

75. Providing tracheostomy care for Mr. Bollela requires that he be suctioned q2h plus PRN. He currently has a No. 6 Shiley tracheostomy tube, uncuffed, with a disposable inner cannula. The respiratory therapist switches on the suction pump on the nightstand, but the pump seems to be failing to deliver sufficient suction. The therapist occludes the distal end of the tubing before attaching the suction catheter and sees the pressure meter climb to only 10 cm H_2O. Which of the following is least likely to be the cause of this problem?

a. dried secretions accumulated in tubing
b. suction canister lid not properly in place
c. clogged in-line bacterial filter
d. system has been recently sterilized

76. The best way for a respiratory therapist to be sure of the concentration of oxygen coming out of an oxygen concentrator is

a. Check the patient's response to an increase in flow rate.
b. Attach the output to an oxygen concentration meter.
c. Listen for the smooth operation of the internal molecular sieves.
d. Make sure it is plugged in properly and that all filters are clean.

77. When the patient exhales slowly into a brand-new, volume-oriented incentive spirometer, the indicator does not move at all. What does this demonstrate?

a. The incentive spirometer is broken.
b. The patient effort is suboptimal.
c. The patient needs a bronchodilator treatment.
d. The patient is using it incorrectly.

78. A patient with tenacious pulmonary secretions has been examined by his physician, who has ordered vibratory positive expiratory pressure (PEP) therapy with respiratory therapist coaching q2h ×5 days. The patient's effort is good, and expiratory force causes the device to vibrate properly. On day two, the patient exhales forcefully but there is no vibration. What should the respiratory therapist <u>NOT</u> do?

a. Check the settings on the device.
b. Determine if the device has accumulated secretions inside of it.
c. Begin chest physical therapy (CPT).
d. Ask the patient to try a few more times.

79. The nitric oxide (NO) delivery device is giving a low-priority alarm, indicating there is a monitoring failure. Which of the following will help troubleshoot the alarm without disconnecting the patient from the device?

a. Close one of the cylinder valves.
b. Check the patient sample line for possible occlusions.
c. Install a new O_2 sensor.
d. There is no way to troubleshoot the alarm without disconnecting the patient.

80. A patient had a chest tube inserted in the ED following a motorcycle accident that resulted in four broken ribs and a left-side pneumothorax. The Heimlich valve on her chest drainage tube is working properly if

a. It allows air to flow out but not in.
b. It allows air to flow out but not fluid.
c. There is no blood seen in the exudate.
d. There is no way to tell if it is working properly without a CXR.

81. The pulmonologist uses a bronchoscope to examine the airways of a patient with suspected early-stage lung cancer for which the diagnostic imaging has been inconclusive. After use, the bronchoscope is delivered to supply for cleaning prior to the next use. The proper method for preparing the bronchoscope for the next use is

a. sterilization
b. autoclave
c. thorough cleaning with antimicrobial wipes
d. high-level disinfection (HLD) with 0.2% peracetic acid

82. To calibrate an oxygen concentration meter, a respiratory therapist can

a. Turn it on and see if it reads 21% while in room air.
b. Connect it to an air-entrainment device and check the readings to see if they agree with the entrainment settings.
c. Insert a fresh battery and look for an alarm indicator.
d. Compare the readings to a calibrated pulse oximeter.

83. In order to keep the arterial blood gas analyzer working properly, the respiratory therapist may be required to perform regularly scheduled quality assurance procedures. NOT included in these procedures is

a. uploading software updates
b. accurate recordkeeping
c. preventive maintenance
d. using control media for calibration

84. An oropharyngeal airway is used for

a. nonemergency ventilation
b. keeping the tongue from blocking the airway
c. conscious patients with asthma
d. patients with oral trauma

85. The laryngeal mask airway (LMA) is preferred over an endotracheal tube in some circumstances. The reasons do NOT include which one of the following?

a. Insertion is relatively easy.
b. Placement requires no equipment.
c. It avoids tracheal and laryngeal trauma.
d. Materials are always hypoallergenic.

86. Mr. Shimizu has a tracheostomy tube in place for six weeks now since his surgery for laryngeal cancer. He may begin to use a speaking valve on his tube, which will enable him to do which of the following?

a. inhale through his tracheostomy tube and exhale through his trachea and oropharynx
b. inhale and exhale through his tracheostomy tube
c. speak without using his vocal cords
d. eat and speak through the valve

87. Prevention of ventilator-associated pneumonia (VAP) is achieved by observing certain protocols and procedures. Which of the following will NOT help reduce the risk of VAP?

a. incline the head of the bed to 30 to 45 degrees
b. provide oral care
c. spontaneous breathing test daily
d. timely administration of albuterol or DuoNeb

88. Ms. Kwame has passed her spontaneous breathing trials and is ready for extubation. What are the steps for extubation, and in what order are the steps performed?

a. suction, deflate cuff, oxygenate, remove tube, assess patient, supplemental O_2 (if indicated)
b. suction, oxygenate, deflate cuff, remove tube, supplemental O_2 (if indicated), assess patient
c. deflate cuff, oxygenate, suction, remove tube, supplemental O_2 (if indicated), assess patient
d. suction, assess, deflate cuff, remove tube, supplemental O_2 (if indicated), reassess patient

89. The physician who is attending to Mr. Borinkov's respiratory infection wants to evaluate the patient for nasotracheal suctioning to determine if it is indicated and safe. Which of the following is not contraindications for this procedure?

a. myocardial infarction
b. acute facial or neck injury
c. coagulopathy or bleeding disorder
d. age over 65

90. One of the possible complications that a respiratory therapist might encounter while performing postural drainage is acute hypotension during the procedure. Which of the following describes the appropriate steps to take?

a. reposition the patient, administer supplemental O_2, request vasopressors, and resume therapy
b. stop therapy, return patient to the original resting position, and consult the physician
c. stop therapy, administer supplemental O_2, reposition the patient, and resume therapy
d. continue therapy with the patient in the Trendelenburg position, and make a note in the chart

91. High-frequency chest wall oscillation (vest therapy) is a fundamental component of secretion clearance for patients with which of the following?

a. cystic fibrosis
b. asthma
c. emphysema
d. bronchitis

92. Incentive spirometry has been ordered for Miss Fontana to assist with her recovery from abdominal surgery. The goal of this therapy is to help prevent

a. pulmonary edema
b. pulmonary hypertension
c. atelectasis
d. hyperventilation

93. In the ambulance on his way from the scene of a domestic violence incident, a young man is receiving supplemental O_2 at a flow rate of 2 L/min via a simple mask. His SpO_2 on arrival at the ED is 97%. While the trauma team is evaluating injuries sustained by the patient, the respiratory therapist might best recommend

a. switching the patient to a venturi mask at 35%
b. switching the patient to 2 L/min via nasal cannula
c. discontinuing supplemental O_2
d. continuing to oxygenate as is

94. One of the patients in the skilled nursing facility where you work has been having trouble becoming accustomed to her newly ordered CPAP machine. The prescribed therapy is 10 cm H_2O of pressure with humidity. The main complaint, which is becoming an impediment to compliance, is that the full face mask is making the patient feel claustrophobic. What is the best thing a respiratory therapist can do to assist this patient?

a. Offer to supply the patient with a smaller mask such as a nasal mask or nasal pillows.
b. Request that the physician prescribe 2 mg Ativan P.O. 1 hour before bedtime.
c. Decrease the CPAP pressure to 6 cm H_2O as a trial.
d. Tell the patient that she should keep trying and that she will eventually get used to it.

95. Acute respiratory failure requiring mechanical ventilation can be the result of all the following EXCEPT:

a. Sepsis
b. Opiate overdose
c. Left-sided heart failure
d. Pneumonia

96. Which of the following sets of decisions must be made before, or at the time of, initiating mechanical ventilation?

a. invasive versus noninvasive, mode of ventilation, FiO_2, rate, PEEP
b. FiO_2, VT, PEEP, type of sedation, high-rate alarm setting
c. apnea setting, high-pressure alarm setting, low-pressure alarm setting, SpO_2 level
d. consult code status, check for contraindications, obtain consent, intubate

97. Why is pressure-controlled ventilation preferred in some situations?

a. The plateau pressure cannot be lower than the set pressure control level.
b. A higher mean airway pressure can decrease the venous return.
c. Improved gas distribution allows for lower VT.
d. It allows for greater alveolar distension.

98. High-frequency ventilation is sometimes used on pediatric and neonatal patients. A typical high-frequency setting is

a. 100 breaths per minute
b. 200 breaths per minute
c. 450 breaths per minute
d. 900 breaths per minute

99. We are caring for a critically ill patient who is on mechanical ventilation. The ABG results are as follows:

Results	
pH	7.36
$PaCO_2$	46 torr
PaO_2	70 torr
HCO_3^-	24 mEq/L
BE	-1 mEq/L
Mode	Volume Control
rate	14
FiO_2	0.35
V_T	500 mL
PEEP	5 cm H_2O

If the patient is on volume control ventilation, what setting(s) might we recommend changing and in what direction?

a. increase PEEP and VT
b. increase FiO2
c. increase VT
d. decrease VT

100. A man with idiopathic pulmonary fibrosis is proving difficult to ventilate due to low lung compliance. The physician has tried to use volume control ventilation to achieve a specific minute ventilation, but the high-pressure alarm of 40 cm H_2O is regularly going off. We might offer to discuss the following change:

a. Initiate noninvasive ventilation.
b. Increase the high-pressure alarm setting.
c. Decrease the rate, and increase the flow.
d. Switch to pressure-control ventilation.

101. A patient in the ICU is receiving mechanical ventilation. The patient's SpO_2 declines from 97% to 88% over a period of just 20 minutes. The patient's breath sounds are good on the right, but they greatly diminished on the left. The endotracheal tube is at 28 cm at the lip. A stat CXR is ordered. Which of the following is it most likely to show?

a. flash pulmonary edema
b. atelectasis
c. right main stem intubation
d. right-side hemothorax

102. A 55-year-old woman with a 42-pack-year smoking history is currently receiving mechanical ventilation for respiratory failure resulting from bibasilar pneumonia. When the patient shows signs of respiratory distress, an ABG is ordered and shows that the PaO_2 has declined from 70 to 52 mmHg. The $PaCO_2$ is steady at 42 mmHg. The ventilator is on A/C mode, FiO_2 is 0.55, and PEEP is 5 cm H_2O. The respiratory therapist is asked for a recommendation to improve the patient's condition. What is the best recommendation in this situation?

a. increase FiO_2 to 0.65
b. increase PEEP to 10 cm H_2O
c. increase VT
d. increase the respiratory rate

103. Mr. Broadhurst, an 80-year-old male, is receiving mechanical ventilation (A/C mode) during his recovery from septic shock. He appears to be making very good progress. His V_T is 640 mL, his respiratory rate is 12, FiO_2 is 0.40, and PEEP is 5 cmH_2O. Mr. Broadhurst's ideal body weight is 80 kg. These settings provide him with ventilation at the rate of

a. 8 mL/kg ideal body weight (IBW)
b. 6 mL/kg IBW
c. 10 mL/IBW
d. 12 mL/kg IBW

104. A patient is being transported from the ED to the diagnostic imaging department for a stat computed tomography (CT) scan. Monitoring shows a precipitous increase in the patient's heart rate from 81 to 125 bpm. There is a drop in the patient's SpO_2 from 99% to 85%. The first response from the respiratory therapist should be to

a. Use bag-mask ventilation to manually ventilate the patient.
b. Immediately return the patient to the ED for physician attention.
c. Check the ET tube cuff inflation.
d. Perform stat ABG while a registered nurse (RN) obtains a 12-lead ECG.

105. To increase the ratio of the duration of inspiration to the duration of expiration (I:E ratio) from 1:1.5 to 1:2 for a patient on V/C mechanical ventilation, the respiratory therapist can

a. increase VT
b. increase PEEP
c. increase FiO_2
d. increase inspiratory flow

106. Patient-ventilator dyssynchrony can result from a number of factors and will increase the work of breathing (WOB) for the patient. If we notice that our patient is demonstrating excessive effort during breaths, and the P_{AW} as a result shows a dip, we might best

a. increase patient sedation
b. decrease VT
c. decrease PEEP
d. increase inspiratory flow

107. A diagnosis of pneumothorax is suggested by the respiratory therapist in the ED by results of auscultation, observation of tracheal deviation, and CXR analysis. The physician concurs with this diagnosis and decides to place a catheter into the pleural space. Five liters of air is aspirated with no resistance to further aspiration felt. What next step is indicated?

a. placement of a chest tube
b. a follow-up CXR
c. initiation of mechanical ventilation
d. thoracentesis

108. We believe that our patient on mechanical ventilation is ready for their first spontaneous breathing trial. The patient does not tolerate this trial well, and in 15 minutes we must restore mechanical ventilation. Before we try again, we must

a. Suction the airway and administer albuterol.
b. Perform an ABG analysis.
c. Wait at least a few hours, allowing the patient to rest.
d. Check ECG, CBC, and electrolytes.

109. The rapid shallow breathing index (RSBI) of a patient on mechanical ventilation is held by many to be a good predictor of successful weaning. We calculate the index by

a. dividing the frequency by the tidal volume
b. dividing tidal volume by plateau pressure
c. multiplying peak pressure by frequency
d. multiplying PEEP by FiO2 and dividing by tidal volume

110. A patient is recovering from an exacerbation of chronic obstructive pulmonary disease (COPD), chronic bronchitis type, and is having difficulty clearing tenacious secretions. Which of the following therapies will NOT assist the patient?

a. Vibratory positive expiratory pressure (PEP) therapy
b. High-frequency chest wall oscillation therapy
c. Inhalation of nebulized mucolytic
d. Heat and moisture exchangers (HMEs)

111. Mr. Brownstein is an 84-year-old male who has been on mechanical ventilation for three days recovering from bibasilar pneumonia. His comorbidities include early-stage dementia and type 2 diabetes. He will have an increased likelihood of successful extubation and continuing recovery if

a. His antibiotics are discontinued.
b. He does not have a Foley catheter.
c. He is conscious and has a good gag reflex when extubated.
d. He is only moderately stridorous upon extubation.

112. A 32-week neonate is being treated for hypoxic respiratory failure. Nitric oxide (NO) is indicated if the patient also shows evidence of

a. patent foramen ovale
b. pulmonary hypertension
c. heart rate > 100 bpm
d. venous $PaCO_2$ < 65 mmHg

113. Premature infants are frequently born with apnea of prematurity. Sometimes this is a minor problem and resolves on its own over time. The respiratory therapist must look for the following signs to help determine if immediate treatment may be indicated:

a. Apneic episodes are longer than five seconds.
b. Episodes are associated with cyanosis.
c. Maternal age is older than 40 years.
d. Bradycardia (less than 2/3 of baseline for more than two seconds)

114. A mild form of tetralogy of Fallot may be evident in an infant who demonstrates

a. abdominal wall abnormalities
b. a heart murmur and intermittent severe cyanotic spells
c. patent ductus arteriosus
d. signs of meconium aspiration

115. We are working in the ICU, and one of the patients we are caring for is a 28-year-old woman who was reportedly drinking a quart of vodka per day prior to her hospitalization. She is on mechanical ventilation for the second day and is very agitated and unsuccessfully attempting to self-extubate. When we notice this behavior, we immediately consult with the intensivist and ask if he would agree with our recommendation to

a. discontinue mechanical ventilation immediately
b. increase sedation
c. change the ventilation mode to synchronized intermittent mandatory ventilation (SIMV)
d. initiate the use of paralytics

116. Endotracheal instillation of which of these preparations is NOT currently included in respiratory therapy practice?

a. surfactant for neonates
b. saline prior to suctioning
c. epinephrine
d. lidocaine hydrochloride

117. When caring for a patient on mechanical ventilation who has a diagnosis of acute respiratory distress syndrome (ARDS), it is important to be mindful of protecting the lungs from ventilator-induced lung injury. Guidelines include all of the following EXCEPT:

a. maintaining the plateau pressure > 28 cm H_2O
b. maintaining tidal volumes between 4 and 8 mL/kg IBW
c. maintaining end expiratory lung volumes with PEEP
d. keeping the patient's head elevated 30-45 degrees

118. Heliox therapy is used primarily in with patients who have which of the following?

a. obstructed airways
b. pain on inspiration
c. hypercapnia
d. bradycardia

119. The RN in the ICU has asked for the assistance of the respiratory therapist in the assessment of a patient's hemodynamic status. The patient is on pressure support mechanical ventilation. She has a reduced cardiac output and lower blood pressure than earlier in the day. We might suggest that the first therapy to try is

a. diuresis
b. one unit of packed red blood cells IV
c. IV administration of fluid
d. change in the level of sedation

120. Per the physician's order, we are changing the tracheostomy tube for one of our patients. We need to assess the patient, review the chart, and assemble our supplies prior to performing the procedure. Which of these lists include ONLY items always needed for this?

a. O_2 tank, surgical lubricant, unit dose of albuterol, gloves, replacement tracheostomy tube
b. tracheostomy tube tie, drain sponge/dressing, suction catheters, Ambu-bag, surgical lubricant
c. gloves, gown, suction catheters, suction pump machine, nonrebreather mask
d. O_2 tank, nebulizer machine, suction machine, sterile water, normal saline

121. In the pediatric intensive care unit (PICU), one of our patients on mechanical ventilation is producing copious secretions. He has a 6.0 mm ET tube, and we have only size 10 French suction catheters on hand. What do we do?

a. Proceed with suctioning.
b. Go to the central supply for size 12 French catheters.
c. Postpone suctioning for the time being.
d. Use an alternate method of secretion clearance.

122. We begin to suction the tracheal secretions of our intubated patient, but we must stop immediately if we see the patient demonstrate

a. choking/gagging
b. increase in ICP
c. tremors
d. bradycardia

123. Mr. Kovacs has been on mechanical ventilation for slightly more than 48 hours and is doing well. He is now afebrile, and his white blood cell count continues to fall. His physician would like the respiratory therapist to administer a long-acting bronchodilator. Before his hospitalization, Mr. Kovacs was taking Spiriva every day. Which of the following can now be administered as a long-acting bronchodilator?

a. Spiriva via HandiHaler
b. Spiriva via Respimat
c. Spiriva via nebulizer
d. A long-acting bronchodilator is contraindicated in this instance

124. Percussion and auscultation indicate that there is consolidation in the right lung of a 27-week gestational age neonate who is receiving mechanical ventilation. In what position do we recommend the patient to be placed?

a. semi-Fowler's
b. Trendelenburg
c. right side down
d. left side down

125. A premature neonate is being ventilated with high-frequency oscillatory ventilation (HFOV). We should recommend increasing the oscillatory amplitude if the blood gas analysis shows

a. pH greater than 7.45
b. $PaCO_2$ of 62 mmHg or greater
c. HCO_3- equal to 24 mEq/L
d. PaO_2 greater than 75 mmHg

126. Mrs. Murphy has asked her physician why he is prescribing an additional metered-dose inhaler (MDI) for her. She is an asthmatic patient, and in addition to her albuterol rescue inhaler, he is prescribing an inhaler with budesonide to be used daily. What is the physician likely to tell her?

a. The budesonide will calm her so she has no asthma attacks.
b. The new medication will be like another type of albuterol.
c. Budesonide is an inhaled corticosteroid (an anti-inflammatory), which may prevent some asthma attacks.
d. She should just take it so her symptoms won't be so bad if she forgets to take her albuterol.

127. A patient with late-stage COPD has fallen and suffered a broken hip. His physician is reluctant to prescribe certain pain medications such as OxyContin or Percocet without close monitoring mainly because

a. These are opioids and in many cases will suppress the respiratory drive.
b. The doctor is afraid his patient may become addicted to them.
c. There is a possibility of an adverse interaction with the patient's daily Spiriva and Advair.
d. These medications are contraindicated for smokers or former smokers.

128. Annual vaccinations for influenza confer which benefit(s) to those vaccinated?

a. reduce the likelihood of getting the flu
b. will help Tamiflu work better if they get the flu
c. reduce colds and flu because both are viruses
d. offer 100% protection against catching the flu in any given year

129. A patient stumbles into the waiting area of your ED complaining of chest pain. Suddenly, and without further warning, the patient collapses to the floor, unresponsive. All other medical personnel are at that moment tending to a motor vehicle accident victim in the trauma bay. The most important thing for you to do immediately upon determining that there is no heartbeat and no spontaneous respiration is

a. Start bag-mask ventilation with 100% O_2 at 15 L/min.
b. Call for help and begin chest compressions.
c. Get the cardiac defibrillator (the automated external defibrillator [AED]).
d. Call for help and prepare to intubate.

130. Miss Edwards brings her three-year-old child to the emergency room reporting that the child is experiencing sudden-onset wheezing and difficulty breathing. Auscultation reveals that the breath sounds are greatly decreased on the right side. There is no fever or cough. What do we first suspect as the cause?

a. status asthmaticus
b. respiratory syncytial virus
c. right lower lobe pneumonia
d. aspiration of a foreign object

131. The respiratory therapist is assisting the intensivist with the care of a patient who has a rapidly failing cardiac status. The ECG shows supraventricular tachycardia (SVT) and atrial fibrillation while the patient is becoming hypotensive and complaining of chest pain. The physician is likely to ask you to assist with

a. electrical pacing
b. administering diuretic
c. intubation and mechanical ventilation
d. cardioversion

132. When the ventilator patient's status, despite everyone's best efforts, has reached the state where any further medical care is deemed futile, the respiratory therapist may be asked to

a. perform terminal extubation
b. change the ventilator to SIMV mode
c. set FiO_2 to room air and PEEP to 0 cm H_2O
d. talk with the family and check code status

133. When assisting the pulmonologist with a thoracentesis, the respiratory therapist is responsible for which of the following?

a. writing the order
b. assist with the sterile collection of pleural fluid samples
c. documenting the procedure as performed
d. performing the thoracentesis while being observed by the physician

134. Mr. Boris brings his son to the community health clinic for a follow-up on his appointment with the physician regarding the child's asthma. The respiratory therapist meets with the father and son in an educational capacity to discuss disease management. There have been no asthma attacks since the last visit. Which of the following would NOT be a component of the family's asthma action plan?

a. how to use a peak flow meter
b. when it is okay depart from the medication regimen
c. how to know when the child's condition necessitates a trip to the emergency room
d. how to chart and understand the results of flow meter readings

135. We meet with Mrs. Tomashevsky at the physician's request. The purpose of our discussion is to determine if the patient has symptoms that indicate a sleep study would be helpful and to give the physician our recommendations. We will ask our patient about which possible complaints?

a. midday headaches
b. shortness of breath while climbing stairs
c. cough with sputum production
d. excessive daytime sleepiness

136. The physician has met with Mr. Stubs to discuss various issues related to helping him maintain his health and hopefully improve his wellness and quality of life. The physician has asked you to work with Mr. Stubs to assist the patient with smoking cessation. One of the best indicators we can use to immediately determine the strength of the nicotine addiction in Mr. Stubs is to ask him

a. At what age did you start smoking?
b. Do you smoke menthol or nonmenthol cigarettes?
c. Were both of your parents smokers?
d. What is the length of time from waking in the morning to your first cigarette?

137. If we are the respiratory therapist assigned to the hospital's rapid response team for the shift, what responsibility is ours for the entire shift?

a. Do not leave the premises during lunch break without arranging coverage from another therapist.
b. Be prepared by knowing the code status of all patients in the facility.
c. Take charge of the CPR if a patient should code.
d. Provide rescue breaths immediately for a patient who has no spontaneous respirations.

138. Generally speaking, when we administer supplemental oxygen to one of our patients via nasal cannula best practices would indicate adding humidity to the O_2 if the flow rate is at least

a. any flow at all
b. 2 L/min or greater
c. 4 L/min or greater
d. 6 L/min or greater

139. Our patient recovering from an exacerbation of COPD is prescribed 1.25 mg albuterol in 3 ml unit dose via nebulizer q4h around the clock. When we check the medication the pharmacy has provided, the label shows that the unit dose they have sent is 0.625 mg per 3 ml. What should the respiratory therapist do in this situation?

a. Administer two unit doses combined in the nebulizer, and chart what you have done in your notes.
b. Check the original physician order, and immediately call the pharmacy if there is a discrepancy between the order and the medication provided.
c. Skip the scheduled treatment, and put in a call to the physician's answering service.
d. Administer the 0.625 mg unit dose, and assess the patient's response.

140. When we are assessing a patient for use of accessory muscles of respiration, it is best done by

a. watching from across the room when the patient is unaware
b. looking closely for shoulder movement (heaving) and neck muscle movement
c. standing next to the patient with your hand placed gently in the center of the chest
d. careful examination of CXR and results of the peak flow meter

Answer Key and Explanations

1. D: When the patient becomes apneic and subsequently asystolic, the obligation is to report this to the charge nurse as soon as possible. Chest compressions, intubation, and bag-mask ventilation are all under the category of resuscitation, which goes against this patient's wishes as expressed in their "do not resuscitate" code status.

2. B: It is not within the scope of practice for a respiratory therapist to change physician orders or simply ignore or modify them. However, the Combivent and the DuoNeb are identical medications (albuterol + Atrovent) with different names and methods of administration. The respiratory therapist should contact the physician to advise them of the duplication and request further guidance.

3. B: With normal circulation and perfusion, the nail bed will become pink again in less than two seconds. Cyanosis means the nail bed would be bluish. With insufficient blood flow, the nail bed would not "pink up." Anemia has no effect on this particular test unless the anemia is severe.

4. B: The heart rate, respiratory rate, SpO_2, and hematocrit are all normal. Hemoglobin is low. Normal limits are as follows: SpO_2 94–99%, pulse 60–100 bpm, respiratory rate 12–20 rpm, hemoglobin 12–15 g/dL, hematocrit 37–46%.

5. A: This is the concise, standard way to report this information that is most useful for assessing patient and her current status. It is universally accepted as the standard metric to gauge smoking history.

$$(number\ of\ packs\ per\ day) \times (number\ of\ years\ smoked) = pack\text{-}years$$

6. B: The fact that there is a decreased vital capacity (shallow breathing) is all that we know for certain. Some patients will take smaller breaths due to pain after a chest wall injury or after thoracic or abdominal surgery. Also, there are several lung pathologies as well as neuromuscular disorders that can cause a patient to have a shallow breathing pattern. The other answers make conclusions not supported by our observation.

7. D: The wheezing throughout the lung field, even though not very acute, suggests the possibility of the presence of asthma. The association of these episodes with mowing the lawn further supports this as a possible diagnosis. Basic spirometry and the methacholine challenge test will support or rule out the diagnosis of asthma. Although the albuterol inhaler (A) might relieve the wheezing, it will tell us very little about its etiology. A CXR (B) will almost certainly not help us understand the wheezing. A "wait and see" stance might represent a danger to the patient's health.

8. A: The patient is showing the hallmark clinical symptoms of COPD, chronic bronchitis type. Though she is not a smoker, smokers are not the only persons who develop this chronic disease. Family history of COPD and persistent exposure to lung irritants are also thought to be causative. There is not enough information to recommend prescribing specific regimen of medications. Clinical symptoms of pneumonia typically include fever and acute onset. Pulmonary rehabilitation cannot be indicated until the disorder is diagnosed.

9. D: The average normal range for white blood cell count is 4,500–10,000. Pneumonia is an infectious process, and we would expect to see elevated levels of white blood cells, greater than

10,000 WBC/mcL. Bacterial and viral infections will, in most cases, cause an elevation in the WBC count.

10. B: Choices A and D do not include charting the observation. Answer C indicates too high a level of urgency for an observation of "traces" of blood. The appearance of trace blood on the dressing may be indicative of granuloma, infection, or another problem related to the stoma. It is very important for the physician to be notified, but it is not an emergency. It must be documented in the patient chart.

11. A: The patient is hypercapnic and would benefit from NIPPV support to help increase V_T. A CXR must be performed to rule out contraindications such as pneumothorax, or unstable fractures. Choices B and D are insufficient because supplemental O_2 may help but will not resolve the hypercapnia. Intubation is not indicated in a patient without airway compromise, severe distress, or instability. It is too aggressive at this point.

12. B: The patient history and current condition suggest a ventilation/perfusion problem—possibly a pulmonary embolism. This is seen by computing the P_a and P_A difference. The clotting disorder points in the direction of possible PE. The other tests are unlikely or unable to demonstrate the presence or absence of a pulmonary embolism.

13. A: When an oxygen saturation alarm is triggered, the patient must first be assessed, as pulse oximetry requires specific contact with the skin and often becomes inaccurate due to patient movement, hair on the skin, patient diaphoresis, or sensor connections. Assess the patient for signs of respiratory distress and check the site of the pulse oximetry probe. If this patient were to be demonstrating signs of distress, the next step would be to suction the tracheostomy tube.

14. A: These results show the slightly increased acidity with a high level of CO_2 partially compensated by an elevated HCO_3. "Acute" is indicated by the decreased $PaCO_2$. "Chronic" is indicated by the elevated HCO_3. The other answers do not show both of these features.

15. D: None of the other tests can measure FRC. FRC can be computed only once the total lung capacity is known, measured either by nitrogen washout or by body plethysmography.

16. D: The other choices are too small to be considered significant. This is the percentage value established by best practices.

17. B: The measurements are all within the acceptable error of ≤105 mL.

18. D: The range for staging of moderate COPD is 50–79%. There is no indication for a CXR (A). The respiratory therapist would be responsible for observing and noting whether or not patient effort was acceptable (B).

19. D: The trachea will deviate away from the side with the tension pneumothorax. The other answers are not indicated by the tracheal deviation.

20. C: Prior to collecting an ABG, the order must be written and reviewed and patient identity must be confirmed with two unique patient identifiers. Next, hand hygiene must be performed before conducting an Allen's test to confirm perfusion, then again hands are washed before donning gloves, preparing the kit, cleaning the site, and drawing the sample.

21. A: Cigarette smoking will increase the level of carbon monoxide in the bloodstream, and this will cause the reading to be incorrectly too high. The CO bound to the hemoglobin will be read as O_2.

Option B is relevant only if the patient is coming directly from a fire. The hemoglobin level (C) is within normal limits. The dark nail polish (D), if it impacts the reading, may give a reduced value. In this situation, we can remove the nail polish or use an ear probe.

22. A: The FEV_1 values show considerable variations indicating an unusable data set. Useful analysis cannot be made.

23. A: Tuberculosis isolation is considered airborne. Answers b and c are insufficient PPE. Answer d includes booties and bonnet required for a sterile environment, but they are not required here.

24. B: Choice A would put our patient still in the green zone. Choices C and D would require a trip to her healthcare provider immediately.

25. D: A recent respiratory infection in an otherwise healthy young person is not a contraindication for pulmonary function testing.

26. A: Choices B and C indicate good curves and good results. A diminished value for FVC1 could indicate COPD, chronic bronchitis, emphysema, or bronchiectasis.

27. A: This is the critical measurement for the respiratory status of a patient with this disease. The other answers may or may not be indicated at other times, but they do not apply here.

28. C: None of the other answers indicate a problem that would give such a result.

29. D: Sputum will not always need to be cultured, but it should always be examined for color, odor, consistency, and quantity.

30. A: Vomiting expels stomach acid and therefore lowers the body's acidity, raising pH. Choice B, hypoventilation, will increase acidity (lower pH). Blood loss (C) and internal bleeding (D) have no predictable effect upon pH.

31. C: The ABG analysis is more reliable than the pulse oximeter in the absence of any signs of hypoxemia. We can follow up with a check of the pulse oximetry apparatus and, if requested by the physician, repeat the ABG.

32. A: End-tidal CO_2 is a very useful measure of CO_2 in the blood; the only other useful (and superior) measure would be sending the patient out for an ABG test. The results of a venous blood draw are not as accurate of a measure and therefore not as useful.

33. B: The sleep lab <u>does not</u> routinely monitor blood glucose (A) nor galvanic skin response (C) nor airway resistance (D).

34. C: This is the defined parameters of apnea hypopnea index for moderate sleep apnea, an average of 15 to 30 episodes per hour. These are the standards of the American Thoracic Society and the Academy of Sleep Medicine.

35. D: Patients at the extremes of weight, patients with high levels of stress, and patients who are difficult to wean from the ventilator are all among the standard indications for a metabolic study with indirect calorimetry.

36. D: The other three observations/reactions are all included in the computation of the Apgar score.

37. B: This is the standard established by the American Medical Association.

38. A: Hypovolemia is the most likely cause. Absent any contraindications, this is the most likely therapy to pursue. Vasopressors may increase blood pressure but not cardiac output. Inotropic agents will increase the strength of the heartbeat but probably not sufficiently if the fluid level is low. Diuretics will have the reverse of the effects we want, lowering the fluid in the body.

39. A: Auscultation will probably show crackles. We know he is not in bronchospasm because we see no indications of restriction in his large airways and no history of a disorder that would cause this.

40. D: Increased respiratory rate, accessory muscle use, and diagnosis with idiopathic pulmonary fibrosis (IPF) are all clinical indications of increased WOB that we can observe. IPF is a disease causing "stiff lungs," which increase WOB.

41. C: These are the parameters we use to define "safe" ICP.

42. A: Hypertension has been associated with the development of a first-degree AV block, which is a regular rhythm with a prolonged PR interval which is one that is >0.20 seconds. Dehydration and internal bleeding both result in hypovolemia which manifests as sinus tachycardia.

43. B: All other values are not within normal limits.

44. C: An obtunded patient is not aware and/or not communicating. Pain is not assessed as far as mental status evaluation. "Orientation to recent events" is occasionally included in the ED or by paramedics and is included in "A & O x4."

45. D: This is the standard method for asking patients to assess their pain. We can use a chart with images of faces to indicate the extremes of pain and the intermediate levels if the patient is nonverbal.

46. C: Clear or white or pale yellow sputum usually indicates the absence of infection. Dark and colored sputum, including traces of blood or frank blood or not, can help with the diagnosis.

47. A: A work environment that has airborne particles, smoke, soot, or chemical vapors can cause many people to experience asthma or asthma-like symptoms. The other questions are possibly of some value in an assessment but not to the same extent with regard to respiratory status.

48. C: Our patient's ability to perform such simple but active tasks will tell us much about her ability to care for herself and the extent of her limitations. We cannot draw accurate and reliable conclusions without such reports from patient experiences (A and B). Observations by family members are valuable but not to the same extent.

49. C: While family and personal history are important to discuss, asking specific questions about the patient's presenting problem (in this case, air quality in the home) is important to determining etiology and a diagnosis.

50. A: Choices B and C include conditions that do not cause tracheal deviation. Atelectasis may cause tracheal deviation if it involves the collapse of a lung or a lobe; pulmonary edema will not. In Choice D, the foreign body aspiration may cause a tracheal deviation if it leads to a collapsed lung but the pericardial effusions will not.

51. C: A lateral neck X-ray will likely show the steeple sign in the throat. The other disorders will not be revealed on the X-ray.

52. D: Lung apices, costophrenic angles, and hemidiaphragms must all be seen clearly on the CXR for it to be a valid study.

53. A: The light area depicts an area of higher density in the anatomy (the pleural fluid). The fluid accumulates first in the costophrenic angle in an upright CXR. The ground glass opacity and the Kerley B lines are findings that indicate the possible presence of acute respiratory distress syndrome (ARDS) and congestive heart failure (CHF), respectively.

54. B: The heart appears larger in the A/P CXR because in this position the heart is closer to the X-ray beam and further from the plate.

55. A: The enlarged liver will exert upward pressure on the right hemidiaphragm. The other disorders will have no effect on the diaphragm.

56. A: The 12-lead ECG yields a great quantity of quality diagnostic information. It is noninvasive and painless. The tracing may or may not be predictive of anything. Limb-leads in the 12-lead ECG may cause artifacts due to patient movement, which are reduced in 3- and 5- lead ECGs because they don't use leads on limbs.

57. A: Minute ventilation (V_E) is defined as the tidal volume (in milliliters or liters) times the respiratory rate (in respirations per minute) $V_E = V_T \times R$.

58. A: When the plateau pressure (P_{PLAT}) is measured and tracked, it can warn of reducing lung compliance. A lower P_{PLAT} measurement is associated with fewer instances of lung injury, and the reverse is also true. Higher pressures are likely to induce injury.

59. D: The concentration of O_2 in the alveoli is equivalent to the FiO_2. The ABG results will show the PaO_2. These two numbers enable us to compute the alveolar-arterial tension difference, and they give us information regarding oxygen transport from the inspired air to the blood.

60. D: Angina with exercise, inability or unwillingness of the patient to participate, and uncontrolled diabetes are all among the contraindications for cardiac rehabilitation. Mildly elevated BMI is not a contraindication of CPX.

61. A: The delay in analysis can produce an inaccurate result. The maximum time delay should be less than 15 minutes. Expelling air bubbles and not aspirating the sample are things that must be done for a good sample collection. Oxygen delivery system and flow rate should be noted, if present.

62. D: The manometer is a pressure-measuring device. Overinflating the cuff (excess pressure) can damage the trachea by restricting blood flow to the lining tissue. Underinflation will impede or prevent proper ventilation and monitoring.

63. B: Hypertonic saline will create osmotic pressure and draw more fluid into the patient's airways. This creates a greater quantity of sputum and makes it easier to cough up. Choices A and C will assist in the general hydration of the patient but may not thin the secretions sufficiently or quickly. Albuterol will likely have no effect on the patient's ability to retrieve a sputum sample.

64. D: Auto-PEEP can be caused by air trapping and the inability to completely empty the lungs. All of the choices EXCEPT diuresis will reduce the likelihood of auto-PEEP.

65. D: Transcutaneous monitoring requires these clinical observations and parameters be charted as a record of the conditions under which the data was collected and for the useful analysis of that data.

66. A: Desaturations shown on the overnight pulse oximetry demonstrate sleep-disordered breathing, and patients who are simply snoring will have no such desaturations. These desaturations are among the key clinical manifestations of sleep apnea. The procedure does not give any indications with regard to the cause (C), nor does it monitor muscle use (B). The Epworth Sleepiness Scale may or may not have been properly administered.

67. B: This is the only parameter included in these options that does not require conscious patient participation.

68. A: The auto-CPAP machine will track parameters and yield useful information whether used in the sleep lab or at home. Experimentation with various settings at home is of little use.

69. D: Hypertension would not cause the results of hemoximetry to be inaccurate and unreliable. Because hemoximetry measures the oxygen-carrying capacity of hemoglobin, it may be inaccurate in the setting of dysfunctional red blood cells such as sickle cell anemia. A dirty cuvette chamber results in a higher than accurate reading of total hemoglobin and hemoglobin that is carrying oxygen. Hyperlipidemia can interfere with the membrane that analyzes the blood and result in false readings.

70. C: The symptoms displayed indicate possible tuberculosis. Central Africa is a part of the world where tuberculosis is present in the population. Of these tests, the PPD test is the one that is diagnostic for this disease.

71. A: Equipment past its expiration date should never be used on a patient.

72. C: Only use machines that indicate that they have been maintained properly by the facility's biomedical technicians.

73. C: The bag-mask ventilation device (Ambu-bag) is required in every room with a patient on mechanical ventilation because it may be used if the ventilator fails or if the patient goes into a crisis. It may also be used during transport to another area of the hospital if this becomes necessary. The other items are unlikely to be of any use.

74. B: Biting on the ET tube can cause great resistance to ventilation. Sedation will not cause an increase in the pressures needed to ventilate; Choices C and D will lower the pressures needed.

75. D: Dried secretions accumulated in tubing, a suction canister lid not properly in place, and a clogged in-line bacterial filter are all possible causes of a decrease in available suction.

76. B: This is the safe quality control measure. None of the other answers will yield an accurate answer to the question of the concentration of O_2. Testing the concentration using a patient reaction to titration is dangerous.

77. D: The patient should be inhaling, not exhaling. Therefore, none of the answers point to the problem or its solution.

78. C: The respiratory therapist may not begin CPT without a physician's order. Initiating this therapy without an order is outside the scope of practice. The other choices are all good options.

79. B: Checking the sample line can be done with the patient still connected; occlusion of this line is a possible cause when troubleshooting for this alarm.

80. A: The drainage tube must not allow air back into the chest cavity. It should allow fluid to drain out. Blood in the exudate does not indicate that the valve is not working properly. A CXR is usually not needed for this determination.

81. D: The bronchoscope does not require complete sterilization or autoclave treatment, but it does need better cleaning and disinfection than can be provided by using antimicrobial wipes.

82. A: This is the simplest test, and it gives reliable results.

83. A: Software updates should be performed by the biomechanical engineers who service the machine. The other answers are items that the respiratory therapist is likely to be required to address.

84. B: An oropharyngeal airway is used in emergency situations only for the purpose of maintaining a patent airway and should not be used if a patient has oral trauma.

85. D: All of the materials used for ventilation and airway management are composed of hypoallergenic materials, with rare exceptions. Choices A, B, and C are all reasons that the LMA is used.

86. A: The speaking valve (or PMV) allows the patient to exhale through the larynx and past his vocal cords to enable him to produce speech.

87. D: Inclining the head of the bed to 30 or 45 degrees, providing oral care, and conducting a spontaneous breathing test daily are all items found on the list of things to do to prevent VAP. Administration of inhaled corticosteroids (ICSs), such as albuterol or DuoNeb, has not been shown to reduce VAP.

88. B: This is the order in which these steps must be performed for patient safety and the greatest chance of a successful extubation.

89. D: Myocardial infarction, acute facial or neck injury, and coagulopathy or bleeding disorder are all among the contraindications for this procedure, which also include laryngospasm, irritable airway, and nasal bleeding.

90. B: Acute hypotension is a cause for immediately terminating therapy. This must be charted. The therapy may not be resumed without informing the physician and obtaining his or her approval in writing.

91. A: Asthma, bronchitis, and emphysema do not cause secretions to accumulate in such a way as to require assistance with secretion clearance. Patients with cystic fibrosis experience the accumulation of tenacious secretions.

92. C: Atelectasis will often occur with patients who are recovering from abdominal surgery. Because it is most likely painful to draw a full breath, these patients will take small breaths and not expand their lungs fully (this is called splinting). The other conditions do not result from these smaller breaths.

93. B: The flow rate of 2 L/min is too low for proper use of the simple mask. It is insufficient to flush out the CO_2 from exhalation between inhalations. The flow is adequate and correct, but the delivery device is incorrect.

94. A: The smaller mask is the first thing to try. Patients who feel claustrophobic with a larger mask can often tolerate the smaller masks. Adding sedation (B) is not called for at this point. Changing the pressure to a lower setting (C) is likely to render the therapy ineffective, and these settings cannot be changed without a physician's order. Choice D will not work with a patient who finds that the mask causes great anxiety.

95. C: Sepsis, opiate overdose, and pneumonia can all put a patient into a state of respiratory failure.

96. A: Choice B includes "type of sedation," which may or may not be indicated. Choice C includes "SpO_2 level," which is also not a ventilation parameter (but may be a goal). Choice D includes "obtain consent," but consent is rarely if ever obtained at the time that ventilation is initiated.

97. C: Improved gas distribution allows for lower VT.

98. D: A typical high-frequency setting sometimes used for pediatric or neonatal patients is 900 breaths per minute, or 15 Hz.

99. C: Judging by the pH (acidic) and the $PaCO_2$ (high) levels, the patient is hypercapnic. An increase in tidal volume will decrease CO_2 levels. Choice A includes changing PEEP, which is not indicated. Increasing FiO_2 will have no effect on CO_2 levels. Decreasing V_T will have the opposite of the desired effect.

100. D: Pressure-control ventilation is preferred with low lung compliance and the danger of barotrauma. Choice A is impractical. Choice B is dangerous and will lead to harming the patient. Choice C is an ineffective solution.

101. C: The 28 cm reading is unusually high and leads us to think that the ET tube might be in too far. Typical is 23 to 25 cm. Choices A and B are conditions that would not favor one side over the other, causing breath sounds to be diminished on only one side. Choice D would cause breath sounds to diminish on the right side, not the left.

102. B: Increasing the PEEP would most likely improve oxygenation without imposing the side effects of oxygen toxicity that might result from a higher FiO_2. Higher V_T and higher rate do not improve oxygenation.

103. A: Calculate this by dividing the V_T (in mL) by the IBW (in kg).

104. A: Tachycardia and an acute drop in SpO_2 indicate the possibility of acute respiratory failure. Begin bag-mask ventilation with 100% O_2 immediately and then return patient to ED physician for attention.

105. D: Increasing the inspiratory flow will decrease the inspiratory time and thereby shift this ratio in the direction we want.

106. D: In this situation, increasing the inspiratory flow will allow the patient to take breaths with less WOB. The need for a higher flow is indicated by the drop in airway pressure (P_{AW}).

107. A: This result from the placement of a catheter indicates that there is air continuing to flow into the pleural space from the lung. The next procedure that is indicated is placement of a chest tube while the medical team tries to reinflate the lung.

108. C: We will not get another meaningful trial without allowing the patient to recover from the exertion and fatigue of the first trial. A second trial following too closely after the first is going to stress and excessively fatigue the patient.

109. A: The formula to calculate the RSBI is respiratory rate / tidal volume = RSBI. Some ventilators calculate and display this number.

110. D: Individually or in combination, vibratory positive expiratory pressure (PEP), high-frequency chest wall oscillation therapy, and inhalation of nebulized mucolytic are all useful therapies for clearing tenacious secretions. HMEs might increase the risk for endotracheal occlusions causing suffocation.

111. C: The patient needs to be able to protect his airway to have a good chance of succeeding post-extubation. The other factors are not predictive of this one way or the other.

112. B: Nitric oxide is a vasodilator for the neonate with pulmonary artery hypertension. Choices C and D are normal values. Patent foramen ovale will require different intervention.

113. B: In the absence of signs of cyanosis, bradycardia (less than 2/3 of baseline for more than four seconds) or observed apneic episodes longer than 10 seconds, we can watch to see if the condition resolves without intervention.

114. B: These are the classic symptoms that indicate this disorder to the exclusion of the others.

115. B: The increased agitation is likely a symptom of alcohol withdrawal, and short-term increases in sedation may be the best course of treatment. Choices A and D are dangerous. Choice B will not solve the problem.

116. B: The practice of instilling saline into the ET tube is no longer used.

117. A: Plateau pressure should be kept below 28 cm H_2O in order to protect against ventilator-induced lung injury.

118. A: Heliox, a combination of helium and oxygen, has a lower viscosity and less resistance to flow through narrow spaces than do O_2 or N_2. Combining the oxygen administered with helium (and not N_2) allows it to flow more easily through restricted airways.

119. C: These are usually signs of hypovolemia, often reversed by administration of IV fluid. Sedation will not help, and diuresis will have the opposite effect. Transfusion of packed red blood cells is not indicated.

120. B: These are the items that must be on hand. We do not need albuterol, the nonrebreather mask, or the nebulizer machine.

121. A: This is the appropriate size catheter to use with this ET tube. Size 12 French is too big. There is no need to postpone suctioning or find another way to clear secretions.

122. D: Bradycardia is a possible adverse reaction to ET tube suctioning. The other choices are unrelated.

123. B: Spiriva is not available in a form for nebulization. HandiHaler is a dry powder inhaler (DPI), which cannot be administered to a patient on mechanical ventilation. The Respimat dispenses a mist that can be administered via ET tube.

124. D: Placing the lung with signs of consolidation up and the healthy lung down is appropriate positioning to relieve pressure on the right lung.

125. B: Increasing the amplitude with HFOV increases the volume of ventilation, decreasing the $PaCO_2$. The other measurements (C and D) are all normal values. A high pH (A) is the reverse of this indication.

126. C: The daily use of an inhaled corticosteroid is commonly recommended for asthmatic patients to reduce or eliminate asthma attacks.

127. A: Great care must be taken when prescribing pain medication to COPD patients. The possible smoking history is not a contraindication, nor do these medications interact with the patient's bronchodilators. The risk of addiction is irrelevant to the COPD.

128. A: This is the definitive benefit of the flu vaccine. The other statements are untrue.

129. B: Once the need for CPR is determined, the sooner chest compressions begin, the better the survival rate. Nothing else is as important as beginning the compressions immediately.

130. D: An aspirated object will most often descend into the right mainstem bronchus, which deviates from the trachea at a less acute angle. Asthma and RSV would affect breath sounds bilaterally, and pneumonia more likely presents with rhonchi rather than wheezing.

131. D: These are symptoms indicating the need for cardioversion as opposed to the other interventions shown. There is disorganized electrical activity in the heart.

132. A: At this point, it is determined that no other interventions are appropriate. The physician's job is to talk with the family.

133. B: Only the physician may order the procedure. The physician documents the procedure as performed, and the respiratory therapist documents the assistance given and other clinical observations.

134. B: Part of the family's asthma action plan would be the importance of compliance with the medication regimen exactly as prescribed.

135. D: This is the single best determinant of whether or not a sleep study is indicated. None of the other answers directly indicate the probability of sleep disorder.

136. D: This is the indicator of the strength of the addiction. The other factors are incidental.

137. A: This is our obligation to our patients and to our team.

138. C: This is where the patient may feel the irritation of the excess amount of dehumidified gas (O_2) being inhaled.

139. B: The respiratory therapist may not administer medication except as ordered by the physician or other practitioner with prescriber privileges. If the order does not comport with the medication sent by the pharmacy, it is the respiratory therapist's responsibility to reconcile this to facilitate administering appropriate care to the patient.

140. B: These are the accessory muscles most commonly used. Careful observation is how we determine if these muscles are being used.

Clinical Simulations

Note: Because of the size constraints of our book binding process, only 2 of our 10 clinical simulation examples appear in this book. The remaining 8 simulations can be accessed on our online resources page: mometrix.com/resources719/crtrrt

Instructions

The following ten simulations start with a paragraph that gives preliminary information about a patient. The sections that follow are identified with a capital letter. Each section begins with specific instructions about the number of responses to select. You will indicate your selection, or selections, by placing a mark in the square. After you make your selection or selections, check your answers on the following page. The answer explanations and "Response Development" sections can provide insight and possibly additional information helpful in completing the other sections.

Simulation #1

A 6-year-old female presents to the emergency department with a tight cough, shortness of breath, and copious nasal secretions. The patient has nasal flaring and intercostal and subcostal retractions. While performing the initial patient examination, the following physiologic data are recorded:

Temperature	98.9
HR	145
RR	44
Breath sounds	diminished with faint expiratory wheeze noted
SpO_2	89%
BP	107/71

NOW GO TO SECTION A

Section A: Initial Information Gathering

Which data would be helpful when completing an initial patient assessment?

DIRECTIONS: Select as many as you consider indicated in this section. After making your selections and scoring your answers, it is beneficial to read the rationales and extended scenarios for all answer choices.

- ☐ 1. History of present illness including home medications
- ☐ 2. Past medical history including vaccine administration
- ☐ 3. Family medical history
- ☐ 4. Urine output
- ☐ 5. Consistency of respiratory secretions

Section A: Relevance and Initial Information Explored

1. History of present illness

INDICATED (+3)
It is helpful to gather a history of the present illness as this information helps determine the timeline associated with the patient's symptoms. A thorough history also helps determine the cause of the symptoms and subsequent treatment plan.

A complete medication history is important for patient assessment because it helps the clinician deduce which underlying medical ailments and comorbidities this patient may have as well as allow the clinician to safely choose additional medications without overdosing the patient or causing negative medication interactions.

This patient's symptoms began after a weekend visit to a pumpkin patch and progressively became more severe over the 2 days after the trip. The patient is unable to sleep at night and cannot lie flat without increasing shortness of breath.

This patient takes Zyrtec 5 ml daily for seasonal allergies in the spring. It is currently autumn, and the patient does not take any daily medications at this time. She has an AUVI-Q for her shellfish allergy.

2. Past medical history

INDICATED (+2)
A past medical history helps determine the cause of the current symptoms. Taking a thorough medical history can indicate whether the current episode is allergic, infectious, or hereditary in nature. This information is essential to the diagnosis and treatment of symptoms.

The patient was born at 37 weeks gestation. She has been admitted to the hospital with respiratory symptoms several times per year since her birth. Her mother says that "colds always go to her chest." The patient has a history of seasonal allergies including mold, dust, pollen, and grasses. She also has a history of allergy to shellfish. The patient received the influenza vaccine at her pediatrician's office one month ago.

3. Family medical history

NOT INDICATED (−1)
Although a family medical history can be helpful for diseases that are presumed to be hereditary or in cases where a highly contagious infectious disease is presumed, it is not generally helpful for an acute allergic illness. This patient's respiratory symptoms indicate a possible acute allergic or mild infectious process rather than a hereditary process; however, it may be helpful to confirm if the patient's family has been ill in the past few days.

No family members have been experiencing respiratory symptoms over the past month.

4. Urine Output

NOT INDICATED (−2)
This patient is not currently experiencing symptoms of heart failure or dehydration and therefore does not require urine output measurement and monitoring.

5. Consistency of Respiratory Secretions

INDICATED (+2)

The consistency of respiratory secretions can provide clues about the patient's underlying disease process. In this case, a bacterial infection is unlikely due to the patient being afebrile. If the patient had a high fever and green or purulent secretions, an infection is the likely cause of the symptoms. If the secretions are clear and the patient is afebrile, an allergic episode or mild viral infection is likely.

The patient has a nonproductive cough and has copious amounts of clear nasal discharge.

RESPONSE DEVELOPMENT:

In summary, the patient's breath sounds are diminished throughout with a faint expiratory wheeze noted. The patient's oxygen saturation on room air is 89%. This patient's symptoms began after a weekend visit to a pumpkin patch and progressively became more severe over the 2 days after the trip. The patient is unable to sleep at night and cannot lie flat without increasing shortness of breath. The patient was a premature birth at 37 weeks and has a significant respiratory history of hospitalizations. The patient is allergic to mold, dust, and grasses and takes Zyrtec in the spring for her allergies. The patient is up-to-date on all vaccinations, including an influenza vaccination, and no members of the patient's family have been sick recently.

NOW GO TO SECTION B

This page is intentionally blank.

Section B: Decision-Making

The patient is becoming increasingly short of breath with increased intercostal and subcostal retractions and nasal flaring. She appears pale, and her lips are dusky. Which interventions should be administered at this time?

DIRECTIONS: Select as many as you consider indicated in this section. After making your selections and scoring your answers, it is beneficial to read the rationales and extended scenarios for all answer choices.

- ☐ 1. Nebulizer treatment with 2.5 mg albuterol
- ☐ 2. Supplemental oxygen via nonrebreather face mask
- ☐ 3. Nebulizer treatment with 0.5 mg budesonide
- ☐ 4. Establish IV access
- ☐ 5. Oral corticosteroid administration

Section B: Relevance of Potential Information Needing Address

1. Nebulizer treatment with 2.5 mg albuterol

INDICATED (+3)

The first line of treatment for bronchospasm is albuterol via handheld, small-volume nebulizer. The standard dose of albuterol is 2.5 mg but can be reduced by half for infants or patients with a cardiac history. This patient would benefit from bronchodilatation with albuterol 2.5 mg.

2. Supplemental oxygen via nonrebreather mask at 15 lpm

NOT INDICATED (−2)

Although this patient is in need of supplemental oxygen, a nebulizer treatment is a better choice at this time. The patient is short of breath and becoming less physiologically stable. The bronchospasm and oxygenation should be treated simultaneously. Nebulizers are given with 100% oxygen; therefore, additional oxygen delivery devices are not needed at this time.

3. Nebulizer treatment with 0.5 mg budesonide

NOT INDICATED (−2)

Although corticosteroids provide quick relief of inflammation during respiratory episodes, inhaled corticosteroids take multiple weeks of continuous use before any benefit is observed. If the patient was due for a budesonide treatment as part of a home medication regimen, it could be mixed with the albuterol and administered via nebulizer; however, this patient does not take any respiratory medications at home.

4. Establish IV access

INDICATED (+2)

This patient would benefit from IV corticosteroid (such as prednisone) administration and may also require additional fluids due to fluid loss from hyperventilation and respiratory distress. IV access is always required in emergencies, including episodes of respiratory distress.

5. Oral corticosteroid administration

NOT INDICATED (−1)

This patient is breathing rapidly and coughing. The priority at this time is to stabilize the patient and reduce their respiratory symptoms. Although corticosteroids are needed at this time, an IV administration would be more appropriate. Patients who are breathing rapidly have a higher probability of aspiration and subsequent aspiration pneumonia, so they should not take anything by mouth unless it is absolutely necessary. IV administration of corticosteroids is more appropriate at this time.

NOW GO TO SECTION C

Section C: Information Gathering

Immediately following the nebulizer treatment, the patient has an oxygen saturation of 95% and respiratory rate of 36, intercostal and subcostal retractions are noted, and breath sounds are wheezing on inspiration and expiration. The patient's cough is tight and wheezy. The patient states she feels better now.

What interventions should be ordered next?

DIRECTIONS: Select as many as you consider indicated in this section. After making your selections and scoring your answers, it is beneficial to read the rationales and extended scenarios for all answer choices.

- ☐ 1. Arterial blood gas
- ☐ 2. Additional 2.5 mg nebulizer treatment
- ☐ 3. Continuous albuterol nebulizer treatment for 1 hour
- ☐ 4. Chest X-ray
- ☐ 5. Peak flow measurement
- ☐ 6. Chest physical therapy

Section C: Relevance and Initial Information Explored

1. Arterial Blood Gas

NOT INDICATED (-2)
An arterial blood gas is not indicated at this time. This patient has improved after her nebulizer treatment and is not in impending respiratory failure. An arterial blood gas is an invasive and frightening experience for a child and should be performed only when necessary. At this time, all necessary vital signs are able to be monitored noninvasively via pulse oximeter and standard emergency department monitoring devices.

2. Additional 2.5 mg albuterol nebulizer treatment

NOT INDICATED (-1)
This patient does require an additional nebulizer treatment; however, due to the severity of the symptoms and the fact that the symptoms have not subsided significantly, it is a better choice to administer a continuous nebulizer. This patient is still significantly short of breath with low oxygen saturations and diffuse wheezing. Although the patient's oxygen saturation has improved, the oxygen saturation measurement was taken immediately after the nebulizer, which is given with 100% oxygen. Therefore, the patient's oxygen saturation immediately after a treatment will be much higher than if the patient were left on room air for 30 minutes and then the oxygen saturation was measured. The patient's current saturation may be abnormally high due to the recent administration of oxygen via nebulizer.

3. Continuous albuterol nebulizer treatment for 1 hour

INDICATED (+3)
The patient is still wheezing, although breath sounds have improved due to improved aeration from the nebulized bronchodilator. The patient is significantly short of breath despite the nebulizer treatment and is still experiencing low oxygen saturations. Due to these factors, a 1-hour albuterol continuous nebulizer treatment is indicated.

4. Chest X-ray

INDICATED (+2)
At this time, it is important to obtain a chest X-ray to help determine the cause of the episode and the appropriate treatment plan. If the X-ray shows an infectious process such as pneumonia, the treatment will be different than if the X-ray shows hyperinflation due to asthma-like disorders. The patient may be transported to X-ray while the continuous albuterol treatment is administered via bedside oxygen tank.

The patient's chest X-ray shows mild hyperinflation of the lungs with no infiltrates or consolidation.

5. Peak flow measurement

NOT INDICATED (-2)
This patient does not have a confirmed history of asthma, despite frequent hospitalizations for respiratory-related illness. Peak flows are indicated only in patients with asthma or for patients with presumed asthma. This patient has not been diagnosed with asthma.

6. Chest physical therapy

NOT INDICATED (-2)
This patient has diffuse wheezing on inspiration and expiration. Chest physical therapy is not indicated for patients with wheezing. Patients with congested breath sounds such as rhonchi and rales can benefit from chest physical therapy. This intervention includes tapping with rubber palm

cups over the patients' lung fields on the chest and back. This helps break up and expel mucus from the airway. This patient does not have a productive cough and does not have rales or rhonchi upon auscultation.

RESPONSE DEVELOPMENT:

In summary, this patient has undergone a continuous albuterol nebulizer for 1 hour followed by a chest X-ray to determine the cause of symptoms and expected treatment plan.

NOW GO TO SECTION D

This page is intentionally blank.

Section D: Decision-Making

After the continuous nebulizer treatment, the patient is resting comfortably with a respiratory rate of 29, heart rate of 150, oxygen saturation of 100%, and normal temperature. No intercostal or subcostal retractions are noted at this time. Breath sounds are clear to slightly diminished on expiration. The patient is playing board games with her mother and is able to speak in complete sentences without stopping to breathe. The patient's chest X-ray shows mild hyperinflation of the lungs with no infiltrates or consolidation. Which action is the most appropriate to take at this time?

DIRECTIONS: Select the most appropriate action indicated in this section. Check your answer. If your answer is not the one indicated, write down your point value, then choose another answer, and check your score again. Your score from this section will be the numbers added together (e.g., if your first choice was not indicated and had a score of –1, and your second answer choice was the one indicated with a score of +3, your score for this section would be a +2).

- ☐ 1. Discharge the patient.
- ☐ 2. Monitor the patient for 1 to 2 hours.
- ☐ 3. Admit the patient for 24-hour observation.
- ☐ 4. Administer a 2.5 mg albuterol treatment.

Section D: Relevance of Potential Information Needing Address

1. Discharge the patient.

NOT INDICATED (–3)

Although this patient has improved considerably, it is not safe or appropriate to immediately discharge her. The clinician must ensure that the patient's oxygen saturation remains normal on room air and the wheezing and shortness of breath doesn't return.

2. Monitor the patient for 1 to 2 hours.

INDICATED (+3)

This patient's symptoms have resolved, but it is possible that her oxygen saturation may drop now that she is not utilizing supplemental oxygen via nebulizer treatment. This patient's symptoms may also return later in the day. Therefore, it is best to monitor the patient for 1 to 2 hours before initiating the discharge process.

3. Admit the patient for 24-hour observation.

NOT INDICATED (–2)

This patient has improved enough to be discharged as long as the symptoms don't return, and the patient's oxygen saturation stays stable. Admitting the patient is not necessary at this time.

4. Administer a 2.5 mg albuterol treatment.

NOT INDICATED (–1)

This patient has received a large dose of albuterol via both small-volume nebulizer and continuous large-volume nebulizer. Additional doses are not required at this time due to the patient's symptoms resolving after the continuous treatment.

NOW GO TO SECTION E

Section E: Decision-Making

After 2 hours, the patient is still resting comfortably and is playing with her family. The patient walked to the bathroom and back with no respiratory distress or desaturation. Her breath sounds are clear and slightly diminished on expiration. Oxygen saturation is 97% on room air. The patient is set to be discharged. What should be included in her discharge plan for home use?

DIRECTIONS: Select as many as you consider indicated in this section. After making your selections and scoring your answers, it is beneficial to read the rationales and extended scenarios for all answer choices.

- ☐ 1. A prescription for oral corticosteroids
- ☐ 2. A prescription for inhaled corticosteroids
- ☐ 3. Orders for a home nebulizer machine from a home health company
- ☐ 4. A prescription for inhaled bronchodilators via inhaler and spacer
- ☐ 5. Patient education including information on prescribed medications and their administration technique
- ☐ 6. An order for home oxygen via tank
- ☐ 7. Instructions to follow up with her primary physician within 2 days
- ☐ 8. A referral to a pulmonologist

Section E: Relevance of Potential Information Needing Address

1. A prescription for oral corticosteroids

INDICATED (+3)

This patient will require a course of oral corticosteroids to treat the underlying inflammation associated with this reactive airway disease process. The chest X-ray shows hyperinflation, which is indicative of asthma or other bronchoconstrictive disorders such as reactive airway disease. This should be treated with a combination of oral corticosteroids and bronchodilators.

2. A prescription for inhaled corticosteroids

NOT INDICATED (–1)

Inhaled corticosteroids are used as a maintenance drug for patients with respiratory diseases such as asthma and chronic obstructive pulmonary disease (COPD). Because this patient does not have a confirmed diagnosis of a chronic reactive respiratory disease, inhaled corticosteroids are not indicated at this time; however, if the patient continues to have episodes of bronchospasm, especially of a cyclic or seasonal nature, asthma may be the appropriate diagnosis.

3. Orders for a home nebulizer machine from a home health company

NOT INDICATED (–2)

A home nebulizer is not indicated at this time. This patient is 6 years old, which is an appropriate age to begin inhaler and spacer training. The only time a nebulizer is more beneficial than an inhaler is when the patient is so short of breath that he or she can't inhale deeply. This patient is breathing comfortably at this time and will be able to use an inhaler successfully with the proper education.

4. A prescription for inhaled bronchodilators via inhaler and spacer

INDICATED (+2)

This patient will require inhaled bronchodilators to continue to treat this episode of bronchospasm. The benefit associated with the inhaler is its portability, which will be helpful if the patient has to use it at school during recovery. The clinician must educate on its use and watch the patient correctly demonstrate the inhaler technique.

5. Patient education including information on prescribed medications and their administration technique

INDICATED (+2)

All home medications must be discussed, and the clinician must educate the patient on each one. This education can include instruction on inhaler technique, side effects of drugs, drug scheduling, and drug dosing. The patient should be provided ample time for questions, which the clinician will answer. The patient should also be provided with a telephone number or source of further information if it is needed. He or she should also be educated on what a respiratory emergency looks like and be given instructions on what to do if another exacerbation occurs.

6. An order for home oxygen via tank

NOT INDICATED (–2)

This patient has normal oxygen saturation both at rest and with ambulation on room air. No additional supplemental oxygen is required at this time.

7. Instructions to follow up with the primary physician within 2 days

INDICATED (+2)

After a respiratory illness with shortness of breath and respiratory distress, the patient must always follow up with a visit to the primary physician. If the patient doesn't have a primary physician, one should be appointed to her.

8. A referral to a pulmonologist

NOT INDICATED (–1)

This patient does not require a referral to a pulmonologist at this time. A pulmonologist referral would be helpful for patients with a history of persistent, uncontrolled asthma that does not respond to initial therapy. This is not the case with this particular patient. This patient had a sudden, acute respiratory episode that is likely secondary to allergen exposure at the pumpkin patch.

Scoring

Simulation 1

Section	Score	Max
A		7
B		5
C		5
D		3
E		9
TOTAL		29
Passing	22	

Simulation #2

You are called to the bedside of a 69-year-old male complaining of shortness of breath and reduced oxygen flow in his nasal cannula. He states he became short of breath while walking to the bathroom. He is currently sitting on the edge of his bed in the tripod position with accessory muscle use noted. His nasal cannula is set at 4 lpm. While performing the initial patient examination, the following physiologic data are recorded:

Temperature	98.4
HR	104
RR	28
Breath sounds	clear with a faint expiratory wheeze
SpO_2	88%
BP	128/90

NOW GO TO SECTION A

Section A: Initial Information Gathering

Which data would be helpful when completing the initial patient assessment?

DIRECTIONS: Select as many as you consider indicated in this section. After making your selections and scoring your answers, it is beneficial to read the rationales and extended scenarios for all answer choices.

- ☐ 1. Admitting diagnosis
- ☐ 2. Past medical history
- ☐ 3. Family medical history
- ☐ 4. Last treatment time, dosage, and outcome
- ☐ 5. Consistency of respiratory secretions

Section A: Relevance and Initial Information Explored

1. Admitting diagnosis

INDICATED (+2)
It is helpful to check the chart for the patient's admitting diagnosis as this information helps determine the best treatment plan for this patient's shortness of breath and oxygen desaturation. An admitting diagnosis also helps determine if the patient's acute respiratory symptoms are new or ongoing.

The patient was admitted to the medical/surgical floor for chronic obstructive pulmonary disease (COPD) exacerbation with acute respiratory distress and hypoxia.

2. Past medical history

INDICATED (+2)
A past medical history helps determine the cause of the current symptoms. Taking a thorough medical history can indicate whether the current episode is caused by allergic, infectious, or hereditary disease processes. This information is essential to the diagnosis and treatment of symptoms.

This patient has a 40-pack-a-year history of smoking and has a history of COPD. The patient requires continuous oxygen via nasal cannula at 4 lpm to keep oxygen saturations at 94%.

3. Family medical history

NOT INDICATED (–1)
This patient is admitted for COPD, which is the underlying disease that causes the current acute exacerbation. A complete family history is not needed at this time as this patient has a definite diagnosis. If the patient had vague symptoms that required further investigation, a thorough family history would be helpful.

The patient has a family history of hypertension and heart disease; however, he does not have this diagnosis.

4. Last treatment time, dosage, and outcome

INDICATED (+3)
This patient is experiencing an acute exacerbation of COPD with dyspnea. The clinician's first priority is to resolve the exacerbation so that the cause can be ascertained. Prior to administering any medications, the clinician must first determine when the last dose of bronchodilators was given. Then the clinician can follow the physician's order and initiate treatment if needed. If the most recent dose was just administered, the clinician may overdose the patient if another is given now. Therefore, a medication history is required in this case.

The patient receives 2.5 mg albuterol and 0.5 mg Atrovent Q4 and Q2 prn for wheeze. The patient's last treatment was 3 hours ago, and it was administered on time.

5. Consistency of respiratory secretions

NOT INDICATED (–1)
The consistency of respiratory secretions can provide clues about the patient's underlying disease process; however, this patient does not complain of a cough. Although many COPD patients do

experience a productive cough, this particular patient is not experiencing one at this time. Therefore, the evaluation of the consistency of respiratory secretions is not indicated.

The patient has a nonproductive cough. No respiratory secretions are noted.

RESPONSE DEVELOPMENT:

In summary, the patient's breath sounds are clear with a faint expiratory wheeze noted. The patient's oxygen saturation on a 4 lpm nasal cannula is 88%. The patient is tachypneic and dyspneic. He complains of reduced flow out of his nasal cannula. This patient's symptoms began after walking to the bathroom. The patient is sitting in the tripod posture at the end of the bed. This patient is admitted for a COPD exacerbation and does not have a relevant family medical history. The patient receives 2.5 mg albuterol and 0.5 mg Atrovent Q4 and Q2 prn for wheeze. The patient's last treatment was 3 hours ago, and it was administered on time. He requires continuous oxygen via nasal cannula at 4 lpm to keep oxygen saturations at 94%.

NOW GO TO SECTION B

This page is intentionally blank.

Section B: Decision-Making

The patient is becoming increasingly short of breath with increased accessory muscle use and posturing. He is diaphoretic and flushed. Which intervention should be administered at this time?

DIRECTIONS: Select the most appropriate action indicated in this section. Check your answer. If your answer is not the one indicated, write down your point value, then choose another answer, and check your score again. Your score from this section will be the numbers added together (e.g., if your first choice was not indicated and had a score of –1, and your second answer choice was the one indicated with a score of +3, your score for this section would be a +2).

- ☐ 1. Nebulizer treatment with 2.5 mg albuterol
- ☐ 2. Supplemental oxygen via nonrebreather face mask
- ☐ 3. Nebulizer treatment with DuoNeb
- ☐ 4. Inhaled corticosteroid administration

Section B: Relevance of Potential Information Needing Address

1. Nebulizer treatment with 2.5 mg albuterol

NOT INDICATED (−1)

The first line of treatment for bronchospasm is albuterol via handheld, small-volume nebulizer; however, this patient is receiving DuoNeb (2.5 mg albuterol and 0.5 mg Atrovent). Although albuterol is a component of the DuoNeb that the patient is already receiving, the patient does not have a separate order for 2.5 mg albuterol nebulizer treatments.

2. Supplemental oxygen via nonrebreather mask at 15 lpm

NOT INDICATED (−2)

Although this patient is hypoxic, a nonrebreather mask provides more oxygen than the patient needs. A nonrebreather mask provides up to 100% oxygen, which can be harmful to patients with COPD. Many COPD patients retain CO_2. When excessive levels of oxygen are administered to a CO_2 retainer, the patient's respiratory receptors can be impaired, resulting in impending respiratory failure. COPD patients should utilize the lowest liter flow of oxygen possible to keep oxygen saturations at an appropriate level.

3. Nebulizer treatment with DuoNeb

INDICATED (+3)

This patient's inpatient medication regimen includes 2.5 mg albuterol and 0.5 mg Atrovent Q4 and Q2 prn for wheeze. The patient's last treatment was given on time 3 hours ago. Because the patient can get additional treatments every 2 hours as needed for wheeze, it is appropriate to administer a DuoNeb treatment at this time.

4. Inhaled corticosteroid administration

NOT INDICATED (−2)

Although corticosteroids provide quick relief of inflammation during respiratory episodes, inhaled corticosteroids take multiple weeks of continuous use before any benefit is observed. If the patient was utilizing a budesonide treatment as part of an inpatient medication regimen, it could be mixed with the albuterol and Atrovent in a handheld nebulizer. The inhaled corticosteroid should be administered only if the patient was due for that medication because inhaled corticosteroids are not quick acting and would not have any effect on the patient's current exacerbation.

NOW GO TO SECTION C

Section C: Information Gathering

Immediately following the nebulizer treatment, the patient has an oxygen saturation of 97% and a respiratory rate of 20, and breath sounds are clear upon auscultation. The patient states that his shortness of breath has subsided.

What assessment should be performed next?

DIRECTIONS: Select as many as you consider indicated in this section. After making your selections and scoring your answers, it is beneficial to read the rationales and extended scenarios for all answer choices.

- ☐ 1. Arterial blood gas
- ☐ 2. Inspection of oxygen equipment
- ☐ 3. Continuous SpO_2 monitoring
- ☐ 4. Chest X-ray
- ☐ 5. Peak flow measurement

Section C: Relevance and Initial Information Explored

1. Arterial blood gas

NOT INDICATED (–2)

An arterial blood gas is not indicated at this time. This patient has improved after his nebulizer treatment, and he is not in distress or impending respiratory failure. At this time, all necessary vital signs are able to be monitored noninvasively at the patient's bedside via handheld pulse oximeter.

2. Inspection of O_2 equipment

INDICATED (+3)

This patient states that it feels as if his nasal cannula has reduced oxygen and flow output; therefore, the nasal cannula system must be inspected and assessed for any leaks, kinks, or obstructions.

3. Continuous SpO_2 monitoring

NOT INDICATED (–1)

This patient had an acute desaturation episode secondary to a presumed equipment failure. Once the equipment is inspected and the problem is resolved, the patient is not expected to have any further episodes of desaturation; therefore, continuous SpO_2 monitoring is not indicated at this time.

4. Chest X-ray

NOT INDICATED (–2)

A chest X-ray is an important diagnostic tool for patients with respiratory symptoms; however, this patient already has a diagnosis of COPD exacerbation with hypoxia. There is no suspected pneumonia, atelectasis, or other respiratory abnormalities. The patient's acute symptoms are not likely to be the result of a new infectious disease process requiring radiological imaging and assessment.

5. Peak flow measurement

NOT INDICATED (–2)

This patient does not have a history of asthma, and therefore, peak flow monitoring is not indicated. Patients with COPD have chronic, progressive reduction in expired airflow. Peak flow monitoring measures increases and decreases in expiratory flow secondary to asthma. Because COPD patients do not have these frequent and dramatic changes in airflow, peak flow assessments are not helpful.

<u>RESPONSE DEVELOPMENT:</u>

In summary, this patient's acute symptoms are expected to be the result of oxygen equipment failure. The patient states his nasal cannula feels like it has reduced oxygen output. The clinician conducts a full equipment inspection, and no further diagnostic or therapeutic interventions are required at this time.

NOW GO TO SECTION D

Section D: Decision-Making

The clinician inspects the patient's nasal cannula system. The humidifier is bubbling furiously and is emitting a high-pitched sound. The flowmeter is set to 4 lpm, and all connections appear tight. No disconnections are observed in the system. The patient is utilizing eight lengths of extension tubing, all of which are clear and without obstruction. There are no kinks or obstructions observed in the system. The nasal prongs are clean and clear of debris. Which action is the most appropriate to take at this time?

DIRECTIONS: Select the most appropriate action indicated in this section. Check your answer. If your answer is not the one indicated, write down your point value, then choose another answer, and check your score again. Your score from this section will be the numbers added together (e.g., if your first choice was not indicated and had a score of −1, and your second answer choice was the one indicated with a score of +3, your score for this section would be a +2).

- ☐ 1. Dial the flowmeter down to zero, then restart the flowmeter at 4 lpm
- ☐ 2. Monitor the patient for 1 to 2 hours
- ☐ 3. Remove all but two extension tubing lengths
- ☐ 4. Replace the nasal cannula system
- ☐ 5. Change the oxygen delivery system to a venti mask

Section D: Relevance of Potential Information Needing Address

1. Dial the flowmeter down to zero, then restart the flowmeter at 4 lpm

NOT INDICATED (-1)
The humidifier is working properly. There is no indication that the humidifier is not functioning as it is bubbling gently and is not emitting any loud noises.

2. Monitor the patient for 1 to 2 hours

NOT INDICATED (-3)
This patient's symptoms are likely due to an equipment malfunction. Allowing the patient to continue to utilize the presumed faulty equipment could result in injury and/or death. The equipment must be assessed, and the problem resolved, or the equipment should be replaced.

3. Remove all but two extension tubing lengths

INDICATED (+3)
This patient is utilizing too many extension tubing lengths. Although the number of extension tubing lengths can vary among manufacturers, eight lengths of extension tubing is excessive and can result in decreased oxygen output in the system. It is likely that excessive use of extension tubing has resulted in decreased flow to the patient and subsequent hypoxia and respiratory distress.

4. Replace the nasal cannula system

NOT INDICATED (-1)
It is appropriate to replace the nasal cannula system when the equipment failure cause cannot be determined; however, in this case, it is likely that the cause of the failure was the excessive use of extension tubing. Therefore, the nasal cannula system does not need to be replaced.

5. Change the oxygen delivery system to a venti mask

NOT INDICATED (-1)
A venti mask can provide appropriate oxygen concentrations for COPD patients; however, some patients do not tolerate masks well due to claustrophobia. Although not harmful, changing to a venti mask is not helpful in this scenario.

NOW GO TO SECTION E

Section E: Decision-Making

After the clinician removes the extra extension tubing, the patient still complains of reduced oxygen flow through the nasal cannula. The humidifier continues to bubble at a high velocity, and the high pitched sound coming from the humidifier has not subsided. No kinks or obstructions were observed in the system during the clinician's assessment. Which action is the most appropriate to take at this time?

DIRECTIONS: Select the most appropriate action indicated in this section. Check your answer. If your answer is not the one indicated, write down your point value, then choose another answer, and check your score again. Your score from this section will be the numbers added together (e.g., if your first choice was not indicated and had a score of –1, and your second answer choice was the one indicated with a score of +3, your score for this section would be a +2).

- ☐ 1. Replace the entire nasal cannula system.
- ☐ 2. Drain and refill the humidifier.
- ☐ 3. Replace the humidifier.
- ☐ 4. Call a rapid response team to the patient's room.

Section E: Relevance and Initial Information Explored

1. Replace the entire nasal cannula system.

NOT INDICATED (–1)
The humidifier is still malfunctioning at this time. The rest of the oxygen system is free of kinks, obstructions, and debris and is expected to be fully functional. Therefore, a complete replacement of the system is not indicated.

2. Drain and refill the humidifier with sterile water.

NOT INDICATED (–2)
The humidifier's malfunction is likely due to an obstruction or manufacturing defect. Replacing the water with new sterile water is not going to help resolve the equipment failure.

3. Replace the humidifier.

INDICATED (+3)
This humidifier needs to be replaced as it is malfunctioning despite a complete system check and removal of the extra extension tubing. Continuing to utilize the faulty humidifier can be potentially dangerous to the patient.

4. Call a rapid response team to the patient's room.

NOT INDICATED (–2)
A rapid response team can be called to the patient's room only in an emergency situation when a patient needs immediate assistance. The clinician is assessing a minor equipment failure that does not require additional personnel. If the patient had become more tachypneic, hypoxic, or unresponsive, then the rapid response team may need to intervene. If the clinician needed assistance, he or she could call a supervisor, not the rapid response team.

SCORING

Simulation 2

Section	Score	Max
A		7
B		3
C		3
D		3
E		3
TOTAL		19
Passing	15	

Special Report: Anatomical Picture Review

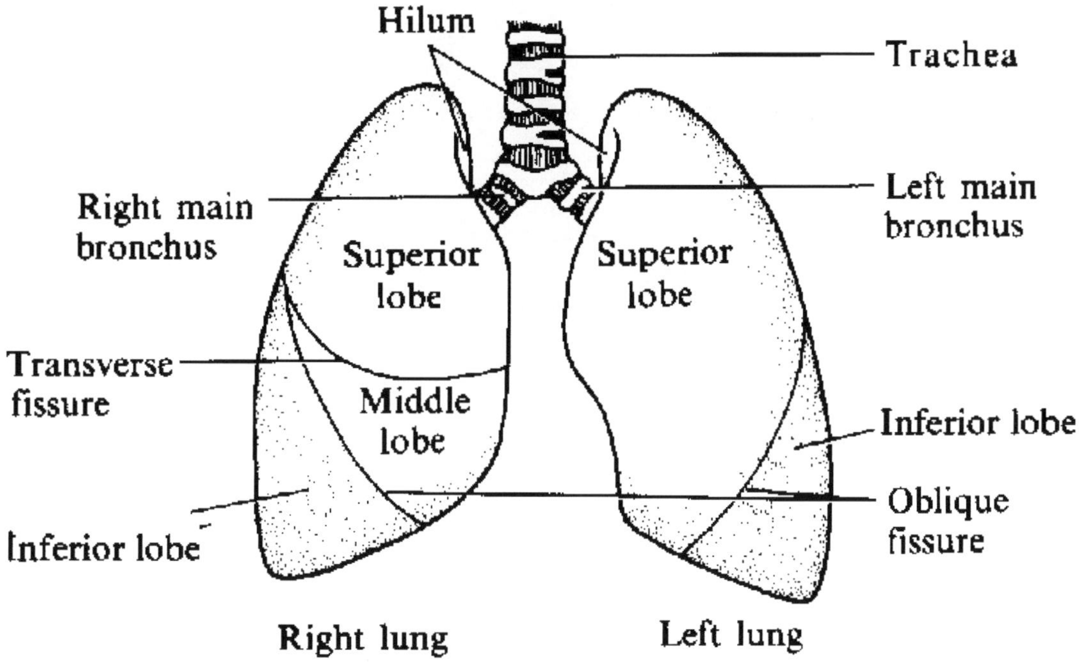

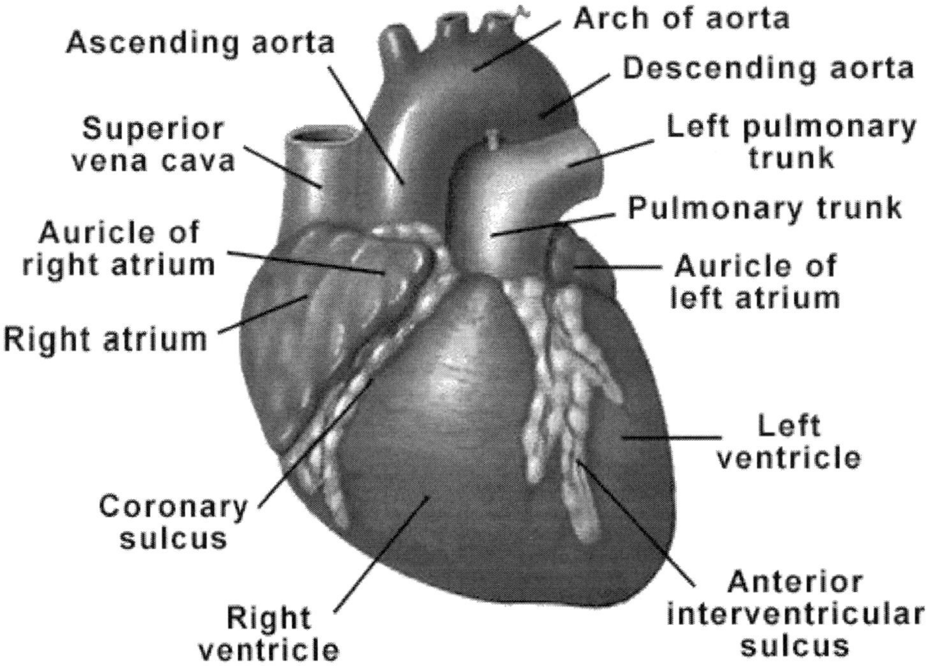
Ascending aorta
Arch of aorta
Descending aorta
Superior vena cava
Left pulmonary trunk
Pulmonary trunk
Auricle of right atrium
Auricle of left atrium
Right atrium
Left ventricle
Coronary sulcus
Right ventricle
Anterior interventricular sulcus

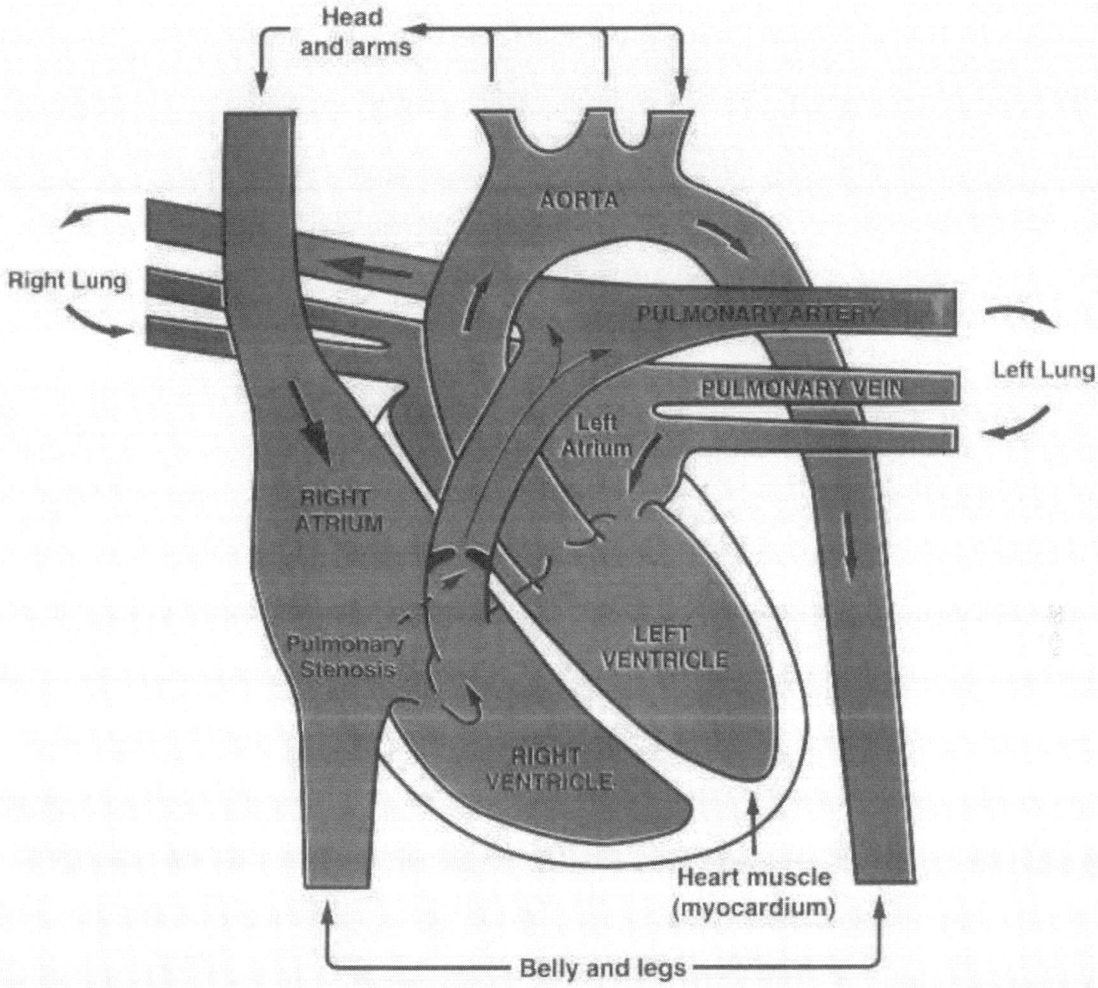
Head
and arms
AORTA
Right Lung
PULMONARY ARTERY
Left Lung
PULMONARY VEIN
Left
Atrium
RIGHT
ATRIUM
Pulmonary
Stenosis
LEFT
VENTRICLE
RIGHT
VENTRICLE
Heart muscle
(myocardium)
Belly and legs

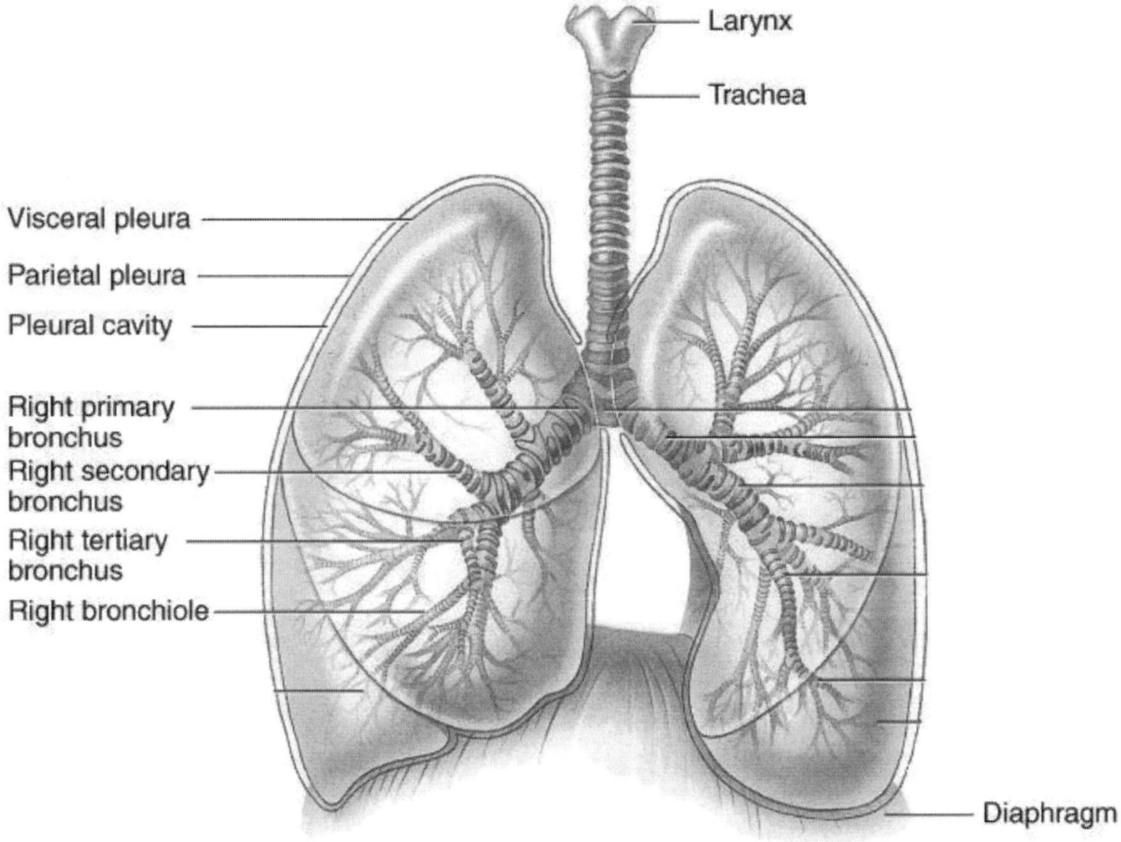

Anterior view

Special Report: Normal Lab Values

Hematologic	
Bleeding time (template)	Less than 10 minutes
Erythrocyte count	4.2-5.9 million/mcL
Erythrocyte sedimentation rate (Westergren)	Male: 0-15 mm/hr; female: 0-20 mm/hr
Hematocrit, blood	Male: 42-50%; female: 40-48%
Hemoglobin, blood	Male: 13-16 g/dL; female: 12-15 g/dL
Leukocyte count and differential	Leukocyte count: 4000-11,000/mcL; 50-70% segmented neutrophils; 0-5% band forms, 0-3% eosinophils, 0-1% basophils, 30-45% lymphocytes, 0-6% monocytes
Mean corpuscular volume	86-98 fL
Prothrombin time, plasma	11-13 seconds
Partial thromboplastin time (activated)	30-40 seconds
Platelet count	150,000-300,000/mcL
Reticulocyte count	0.5-1.5% of red cells
Whole Blood, Plasma, Serum Chemistries	
Amylase, serum	25-125 U/L
Arterial studies, blood (patient breathing room air):	
PO_2	75-100 mm Hg
PCO_2	38-42 mm Hg
Bicarbonate	23-26 mEq/L
pH	7.38-7.44
Oxygen saturation	95% or greater
Bicarbonate, serum	23-28 mEq/L
Bilirubin, serum:	
Total	0.3-1.0 mg/dL
Direct	0.1-0.3 mg/dL
Comprehensive metabolic panel:	
Bilirubin, serum (total)	0.3-1.0 mg/dL
Calcium, serum	Male: 9.0-10.5 mg/dL; female: 8.5-10.2 mg/dL
Cholesterol, serum (total)	Desirable: less than 200 mg/dL Borderline-high: 200-239 mg/dL (may be high in the presence of coronary artery disease or other risk factors) High: greater than 239 mg/dL
Creatinine, serum	0.7-1.5 mg/dL

Glucose, plasma	Normal (fasting): 70-115 mg/dL Borderline: 115-140 mg/dL Abnormal: greater than 140 mg/dL
Phosphorus, serum	3.0-4.5 mg/dL
Proteins, serum:	
Pre-Albumin	0.2 - 0.4 g/dL
Albumin	3.5-5.5 g/dL
Urea nitrogen, blood (BUN)	8-20 mg/dL
Uric acid, serum	3.0-7.0 mg/dL
Cholesterol, serum:	
High-density lipoprotein (HDL)	Low: less than 40 mg/dL
Low-density lipoprotein (LDL)	Optimal: less than 100 mg/dL Near-optimal: 100-129 mg/dL Borderline-high: 130-159 mg/dL (may be high in the presence of coronary artery disease or other risk factors) High: 160-189 mg/dL Very high: 190 mg/dL and above
Triglycerides, serum (fasting)	Normal: less than 250 mg/dL Borderline: 250-500 mg/dL Abnormal: greater than 500 mg/dL
Electrolytes, serum:	
Sodium	136-145 mEq/L
Potassium	3.5-5.0 mEq/L
Chloride	98-106 mEq/L
Follicle-stimulating hormone, serum	Adult male: 2-18 mLU/mL Female: 5-20 mLU/mL (follicular or luteal) 30-50 mLU/mL (mid-cycle peak) greater than 50 mLU/mL (postmenopausal)
Lactate dehydrogenase, serum	140-280 U/L
Osmolality, serum	280-300 mOsm/kg H_2O
Phosphatase (alkaline), serum	30-120 U/L

Special Report: Key Formulas

CARDIOVASCULAR VALUES

Parameter	Derivation	Normal Range
MAP (Mean Artery Pressure)	diastolic + [systolic-diastolic]/3	80-95 mmHg
Pulse Pressure	[systolic – diastolic]	30-50 mmHg
SaO_2 (Arterial Oxygen Saturation)	measured, pulse ox	95-100%
SvO_2 (Mixed Venous Oxygen Saturation)	measured	60-80%
PaO_2 (Partial Pressure of Oxygen - Arterial Blood, Arterial Oxygen Tension)	measured (ABG), [100 - (age - 25)/3]	78-100 mmHg
$PaCO_2$ (Partial Pressure of CO_2 - Arterial Blood, Arterial CO_2 Tension)	measured (ABG)	35-45 mmHg
RAP (Right Atrial Pressure), CVP (Central Venous Pressure)	measured	2-10 mmHg
RVP (Right Ventricle)	measured	15-30 / 0-5 mmHg
PAS / PAD (Pulmonary Artery Systolic / Pulmonary Artery Diastolic) = PAP (Pulmonary Artery Pressure)	measured	15-30 / 8-15 mmHg
PCWP (Pulmonary Capillary Wedge Pressure), PAOP (Pulmonary Artery Occlusion Pressure)	measured	5-16 mmHg
SVR (Systolic Vascular Resistance)	[(MAP – CVP) × 79.9] / CO	770-1500 dynes-sec/cm^5
SVRI (Systolic Vascular Resistance Index)	[(MAP – CVP) × 79.9] / CI	1950-2450 dynes-sec/cm^5/m^2
PVR (Pulmonary Vascular Resistance)	[(MPAP – PAOP) × 79.9] / CO	20-150 dynes-sec/cm^5
PVRI (Pulmonary Vascular Resistance Index)	[(MPAP – PAOP) × 79.9] / CI	50-280 dynes-sec/cm^5/m^2
SV (Stroke Volume)	CO / HR	55-100 ml/beat
SVI (Stroke Volume Index)	CI / HR, or SV / BSA	35-60 ml/beat/m^2
LVSW (Left Ventricular Stroke Work)	SV × (MAP – CVP) × 0.0136	60-105 g-m/beat
LVSWI (Left Ventricular Stroke Work Index)	SVI × (MAP – CVP) × 0.0136	42-62 g-m/m^2/beat

Parameter	Derivation	Normal Range
RVSWI (Right Ventricular Stroke Work Index)	SVI × (MPAP – PAOP) × 0.0136	12-17 g-m/m²/beat
RVEDV (Right Ventricular End Diastolic Volume)	SV / EF	100-150 mL
CaO_2 (Arterial O_2 Content)	[(Hb × 1.34) SaO_2] + [PaO_2 × 0.0031]	16-22 mL O_2 / dL blood
CvO_2 (Mixed Venous O_2 Content, where v = mixed venous)	[(Hb × 1.34) SvO_2] + [PvO_2 × 0.0031]	12-17 mL O_2 / dL blood
$C(a-v)O_2$, or $AVDO_2$ (AV O_2 Difference)	CaO_2 - CvO_2 = (Hb × 1.34) × (SaO_2 - SvO_2)	3.5-5.5 mL O_2 / dL blood
CO, Q_t, (Cardiac Output) – Fick Equation, where V = consumption	SV × HR = VO_2 / [$C(a-v)O_2$ × 10]	4-8 L/min
CI (Cardiac Index)	CO / BSA	2.8-4.0 L/min/m²
DO_2 (O_2 Delivery)	CaO_2 × CO × 10	700-1400 mL/min
DO_2I (O_2 Delivery Index)	CaO_2 × CI × 10	600-800 mL/min/m²
VO_2 (O_2 Consumption)	$C(a-v)O_2$ × CO × 10	180-280 mL/min
VCO_2 (CO_2 Production)		150-230 mL/min
OUC, O_2ER (Oxygen Utilization Coefficient, Oxygen Extraction Ratio)	VO_2 / DO_2	0.23-0.32
RQ (Respiratory Quotient)	VCO_2 / VO_2, where VCO_2 = CO_2 production	normal: 0.75-0.90 pure carbohydrates: 1.0 protein: 0.8 fat: 0.7
CcO_2 (Pulmonary End Capillary O_2 Content)	(Hb × 1.37 × 1) + 0.0031 [0.5(P_{ATM} - 47) -P_ACO_2]	
Q_s / Q_t (Shunt Fraction)	[CcO_2 - CaO_2] / [CcO_2 - CvO_2]	0.05, or 5%

Respiratory Values

Parameter	Derivation	Normal Range
TLC (Total Lung Capacity)	TLC = VC + RV	80 mL/kg, or about 5.0-6.0 L
VC (Vital Capacity)	VC = IRV + ERV + TV	> 75-80% predicted
V_E (Minute Ventilation)	TV × RR	4-6.5 L/min, or about 100 mL/kg/min
P_AO_2 (Alveolar O_2 Pressure, Alveolar Air Equation)	(P_B – P_{H2O}) FiO_2 – [$PaCO_2$ × 1.25], where P_B = 760 mmHg at sea level, and P_{H2O} = 47 mmHg, and 1.25 is the inverse of the RQ	
PaO_2 (Arterial O_2 Pressure)	measured	room air: 80-100 mmHg

Parameter	Derivation	Normal Range
A-a Gradient (Alveolar Arterial Oxygen Gradient)	P_AO_2 - PaO_2 = [(713) FiO_2 - $PaCO_2 \times 1.25$] – PaO_2	room air (21% FiO_2): 2-22 mmHg; 100% FiO_2: 10-60 mmHg
Oxygen Index	PaO_2 / FiO_2	500
VA (Alveolar Ventilation)	[VCO_2 / $PaCO_2$] K	4-6 L/min
VD / VT (VD = dead space, and VT = tidal volume) – Bohr Equation* or Physiologic~	*[P_ACO_2 – P_ECO_2] / P_ACO_2, or ~[P_aCO_2 – P_ECO_2] / P_aCO_2	0.2-0.4
R_{aw} (Airway Resistance)	[P_{alv} – P_{mouth}] / V	1.5-2.0 cm H_2O/L/sec
Compliance	*delta* Volume / *delta* Pressure	
Static Compliance	VT / [Plateau Pressure – PEEP]	50-85 mL/cm H_2O
Dynamic Compliance	VT / [Peak Inspiratory Pressure – PEEP]	75-125 mL/cm H_2O
Chest Wall Compliance	VT / [Airway Pressure – Intrapleural Pressure]	×
Pulmonary Blood Flow Distribution	Zone 1: $P_A > P_a > P_v$ Zone 2: $P_a > P_A > P_v$ Zone 3: $P_a > P_v > P_A$	

Acid/Base Relationships

Anion Gap	Na^+ - (Cl + HCO_3), with normal range 8-12 mmol/L or mEq/L
Base or Bicarbonate Deficit, Metabolic Acidosis (mEq/L)	0.4 (wt in kg) × [desired bicarbonate – observed bicarbonate]
Free Water Deficit	(0.6) × (wt in kg) × [(serum sodium / 140) - 1]; Note - measured in liters, fluid Rx for hypernatremia, infuse 50% of calculated deficit over 1st 24 hours and the remainder over the following 1-2 days
Henderson Hasselbach Equation	pH = pK + log [(HCO_3) / (H_2CO_3)], or pH = 6.1 + log [(HCO_3 / 0.03 ($PaCO_2$)]
Hydrogen Ion Concentration	[H^+] nm/L = 24 (PCO_2) / HCO_3
Rules for Metabolic Compensations for Primary Acute and Chronic Respiratory and Alkalosis	**1.** During acute hypercapnia, HCO_3 increases 1 mmol/L for each 10 mmHg increase in $PaCO_2$ above 40 mmHg. **2.** During chronic hypercapnia, HCO_3 increases 3-4 mmol/L for each 10 mmHg increase in $PaCO_2$ above 40 mmHg. **3.** During acute hypocapnia, HCO_3 decreases 2 mmol/L for every 10 mmHg decrease in $PaCO_2$ below 40 mmHg. **4.** During chronic hypocapnia, HCO_3 decreases 4-5 mmol/L for every 10 mmHg decrease in $PaCO_2$ below 40 mmHg.
Oxyhemoglobin Dissociation Curve and Alkalosis (alkalosis shifts the curve to the left)	Each 0.10 pH rise lowers the PaO_2 about 10%, and oxygen availability to tissues is also reduced by about 10% for each pH increase of 0.10.

Osmolality, Calculated	[2 × Na^+] + BUN/2.8 + Glucose/18 + ETOH/4.6 + Ethylene Glycol/6.2 + Methanol/3.2 + Isopropanol/6.0
Osmolar Gap	Measured Osmolality – Calculated Osmolality; An osmolar gap > 10 mOsm/L suggests the presence of abnormal solutes such as lactate, methanol, ethanol...
pH Changes	1. If the pH rises by 0.10, then K^+ falls an average of 0.5 mEq/L. 2. If the pH rises by 0.10, then ionized calcium and magnesium fall 3-8%.
Parkland Formula (Burn Resuscitation)	4 mL crystalloid / kg / % burn - over 24 hours (50% over the first 8 hours, then 50% over the following 16 hours)
Sodium Bicarbonate Replacement Dose	(base deficit in mEq/L) × (wt in kg) / 4; Note - replace 1/2 of the deficit over 8-12 hours in a non-cardiac arrest situation.
Winter's Formula, Respiratory Compensation for Metabolic Acidosis	$PCO_2 = (HCO_3)(1.5) + 8 \pm 4$

Pediatric Considerations

Blood Pressure - Systolic, age 1-10, 50th percentile	90 mmHg + (age in years × 2) mmHg
Blood Pressure - Systolic, lower limits, 5th percentile	70 mmHg + (age in years × 2) mmHg
Creatinine Clearance	[0.48 × ht in cm × BSA] / [creatinine mg/dL × 1.73]
Defibrillation for Ventricular Fibrillation or Pulseless Ventricular Tachycardia	2 J/kg, then 4 J/kg, then 4 J/kg
ET (Endotracheal) Tube Size (internal diameter - mm)	(16 + age in years) / 4, or [(age in years) / 4] + 4; Note - use an uncuffed ET tube for ages < 8 years.
ET (Endotracheal) Tube Insertion Depth Determination	12 + (age in years / 2) cm; Note - measured from lips.
Fluid Deficit Replacement	[(estimated deficit - %) / 100] × (wt - kg); Note - give 1st half over the first eight hours, and the 2nd half over the next 16 hours.

How to Overcome Test Anxiety

Just the thought of taking a test is enough to make most people a little nervous. A test is an important event that can have a long-term impact on your future, so it's important to take it seriously and it's natural to feel anxious about performing well. But just because anxiety is normal, that doesn't mean that it's helpful in test taking, or that you should simply accept it as part of your life. Anxiety can have a variety of effects. These effects can be mild, like making you feel slightly nervous, or severe, like blocking your ability to focus or remember even a simple detail.

If you experience test anxiety—whether severe or mild—it's important to know how to beat it. To discover this, first you need to understand what causes test anxiety.

Causes of Test Anxiety

While we often think of anxiety as an uncontrollable emotional state, it can actually be caused by simple, practical things. One of the most common causes of test anxiety is that a person does not feel adequately prepared for their test. This feeling can be the result of many different issues such as poor study habits or lack of organization, but the most common culprit is time management. Starting to study too late, failing to organize your study time to cover all of the material, or being distracted while you study will mean that you're not well prepared for the test. This may lead to cramming the night before, which will cause you to be physically and mentally exhausted for the test. Poor time management also contributes to feelings of stress, fear, and hopelessness as you realize you are not well prepared but don't know what to do about it.

Other times, test anxiety is not related to your preparation for the test but comes from unresolved fear. This may be a past failure on a test, or poor performance on tests in general. It may come from comparing yourself to others who seem to be performing better or from the stress of living up to expectations. Anxiety may be driven by fears of the future—how failure on this test would affect your educational and career goals. These fears are often completely irrational, but they can still negatively impact your test performance.

Elements of Test Anxiety

As mentioned earlier, test anxiety is considered to be an emotional state, but it has physical and mental components as well. Sometimes you may not even realize that you are suffering from test anxiety until you notice the physical symptoms. These can include trembling hands, rapid heartbeat, sweating, nausea, and tense muscles. Extreme anxiety may lead to fainting or vomiting. Obviously, any of these symptoms can have a negative impact on testing. It is important to recognize them as soon as they begin to occur so that you can address the problem before it damages your performance.

The mental components of test anxiety include trouble focusing and inability to remember learned information. During a test, your mind is on high alert, which can help you recall information and stay focused for an extended period of time. However, anxiety interferes with your mind's natural processes, causing you to blank out, even on the questions you know well. The strain of testing during anxiety makes it difficult to stay focused, especially on a test that may take several hours. Extreme anxiety can take a huge mental toll, making it difficult not only to recall test information but even to understand the test questions or pull your thoughts together.

Effects of Test Anxiety

Test anxiety is like a disease—if left untreated, it will get progressively worse. Anxiety leads to poor performance, and this reinforces the feelings of fear and failure, which in turn lead to poor performances on subsequent tests. It can grow from a mild nervousness to a crippling condition. If allowed to progress, test anxiety can have a big impact on your schooling, and consequently on your future.

Test anxiety can spread to other parts of your life. Anxiety on tests can become anxiety in any stressful situation, and blanking on a test can turn into panicking in a job situation. But fortunately, you don't have to let anxiety rule your testing and determine your grades. There are a number of relatively simple steps you can take to move past anxiety and function normally on a test and in the rest of life.

Physical Steps for Beating Test Anxiety

While test anxiety is a serious problem, the good news is that it can be overcome. It doesn't have to control your ability to think and remember information. While it may take time, you can begin taking steps today to beat anxiety.

Just as your first hint that you may be struggling with anxiety comes from the physical symptoms, the first step to treating it is also physical. Rest is crucial for having a clear, strong mind. If you are tired, it is much easier to give in to anxiety. But if you establish good sleep habits, your body and mind will be ready to perform optimally, without the strain of exhaustion. Additionally, sleeping well helps you to retain information better, so you're more likely to recall the answers when you see the test questions.

Getting good sleep means more than going to bed on time. It's important to allow your brain time to relax. Take study breaks from time to time so it doesn't get overworked, and don't study right before bed. Take time to rest your mind before trying to rest your body, or you may find it difficult to fall asleep.

Along with sleep, other aspects of physical health are important in preparing for a test. Good nutrition is vital for good brain function. Sugary foods and drinks may give a burst of energy but this burst is followed by a crash, both physically and emotionally. Instead, fuel your body with protein and vitamin-rich foods.

Also, drink plenty of water. Dehydration can lead to headaches and exhaustion, especially if your brain is already under stress from the rigors of the test. Particularly if your test is a long one, drink water during the breaks. And if possible, take an energy-boosting snack to eat between sections.

Along with sleep and diet, a third important part of physical health is exercise. Maintaining a steady workout schedule is helpful, but even taking 5-minute study breaks to walk can help get your blood pumping faster and clear your head. Exercise also releases endorphins, which contribute to a positive feeling and can help combat test anxiety.

When you nurture your physical health, you are also contributing to your mental health. If your body is healthy, your mind is much more likely to be healthy as well. So take time to rest, nourish your body with healthy food and water, and get moving as much as possible. Taking these physical steps will make you stronger and more able to take the mental steps necessary to overcome test anxiety.

Mental Steps for Beating Test Anxiety

Working on the mental side of test anxiety can be more challenging, but as with the physical side, there are clear steps you can take to overcome it. As mentioned earlier, test anxiety often stems from lack of preparation, so the obvious solution is to prepare for the test. Effective studying may be the most important weapon you have for beating test anxiety, but you can and should employ several other mental tools to combat fear.

First, boost your confidence by reminding yourself of past success—tests or projects that you aced. If you're putting as much effort into preparing for this test as you did for those, there's no reason you should expect to fail here. Work hard to prepare; then trust your preparation.

Second, surround yourself with encouraging people. It can be helpful to find a study group, but be sure that the people you're around will encourage a positive attitude. If you spend time with others who are anxious or cynical, this will only contribute to your own anxiety. Look for others who are motivated to study hard from a desire to succeed, not from a fear of failure.

Third, reward yourself. A test is physically and mentally tiring, even without anxiety, and it can be helpful to have something to look forward to. Plan an activity following the test, regardless of the outcome, such as going to a movie or getting ice cream.

When you are taking the test, if you find yourself beginning to feel anxious, remind yourself that you know the material. Visualize successfully completing the test. Then take a few deep, relaxing breaths and return to it. Work through the questions carefully but with confidence, knowing that you are capable of succeeding.

Developing a healthy mental approach to test taking will also aid in other areas of life. Test anxiety affects more than just the actual test—it can be damaging to your mental health and even contribute to depression. It's important to beat test anxiety before it becomes a problem for more than testing.

Study Strategy

Being prepared for the test is necessary to combat anxiety, but what does being prepared look like? You may study for hours on end and still not feel prepared. What you need is a strategy for test prep. The next few pages outline our recommended steps to help you plan out and conquer the challenge of preparation.

Step 1: Scope Out the Test

Learn everything you can about the format (multiple choice, essay, etc.) and what will be on the test. Gather any study materials, course outlines, or sample exams that may be available. Not only will this help you to prepare, but knowing what to expect can help to alleviate test anxiety.

Step 2: Map Out the Material

Look through the textbook or study guide and make note of how many chapters or sections it has. Then divide these over the time you have. For example, if a book has 15 chapters and you have five days to study, you need to cover three chapters each day. Even better, if you have the time, leave an extra day at the end for overall review after you have gone through the material in depth.

If time is limited, you may need to prioritize the material. Look through it and make note of which sections you think you already have a good grasp on, and which need review. While you are studying, skim quickly through the familiar sections and take more time on the challenging parts.

Write out your plan so you don't get lost as you go. Having a written plan also helps you feel more in control of the study, so anxiety is less likely to arise from feeling overwhelmed at the amount to cover.

Step 3: Gather Your Tools

Decide what study method works best for you. Do you prefer to highlight in the book as you study and then go back over the highlighted portions? Or do you type out notes of the important information? Or is it helpful to make flashcards that you can carry with you? Assemble the pens, index cards, highlighters, post-it notes, and any other materials you may need so you won't be distracted by getting up to find things while you study.

If you're having a hard time retaining the information or organizing your notes, experiment with different methods. For example, try color-coding by subject with colored pens, highlighters, or post-it notes. If you learn better by hearing, try recording yourself reading your notes so you can listen while in the car, working out, or simply sitting at your desk. Ask a friend to quiz you from your flashcards, or try teaching someone the material to solidify it in your mind.

Step 4: Create Your Environment

It's important to avoid distractions while you study. This includes both the obvious distractions like visitors and the subtle distractions like an uncomfortable chair (or a too-comfortable couch that makes you want to fall asleep). Set up the best study environment possible: good lighting and a comfortable work area. If background music helps you focus, you may want to turn it on, but otherwise keep the room quiet. If you are using a computer to take notes, be sure you don't have any other windows open, especially applications like social media, games, or anything else that could distract you. Silence your phone and turn off notifications. Be sure to keep water close by so you stay hydrated while you study (but avoid unhealthy drinks and snacks).

Also, take into account the best time of day to study. Are you freshest first thing in the morning? Try to set aside some time then to work through the material. Is your mind clearer in the afternoon or evening? Schedule your study session then. Another method is to study at the same time of day that you will take the test, so that your brain gets used to working on the material at that time and will be ready to focus at test time.

Step 5: Study!

Once you have done all the study preparation, it's time to settle into the actual studying. Sit down, take a few moments to settle your mind so you can focus, and begin to follow your study plan. Don't give in to distractions or let yourself procrastinate. This is your time to prepare so you'll be ready to fearlessly approach the test. Make the most of the time and stay focused.

Of course, you don't want to burn out. If you study too long you may find that you're not retaining the information very well. Take regular study breaks. For example, taking five minutes out of every hour to walk briskly, breathing deeply and swinging your arms, can help your mind stay fresh.

As you get to the end of each chapter or section, it's a good idea to do a quick review. Remind yourself of what you learned and work on any difficult parts. When you feel that you've mastered the material, move on to the next part. At the end of your study session, briefly skim through your notes again.

But while review is helpful, cramming last minute is NOT. If at all possible, work ahead so that you won't need to fit all your study into the last day. Cramming overloads your brain with more information than it can process and retain, and your tired mind may struggle to recall even previously learned information when it is overwhelmed with last-minute study. Also, the urgent nature of cramming and the stress placed on your brain contribute to anxiety. You'll be more likely to go to the test feeling unprepared and having trouble thinking clearly.

So don't cram, and don't stay up late before the test, even just to review your notes at a leisurely pace. Your brain needs rest more than it needs to go over the information again. In fact, plan to finish your studies by noon or early afternoon the day before the test. Give your brain the rest of the day to relax or focus on other things, and get a good night's sleep. Then you will be fresh for the test and better able to recall what you've studied.

Step 6: Take a Practice Test

Many courses offer sample tests, either online or in the study materials. This is an excellent resource to check whether you have mastered the material, as well as to prepare for the test format and environment.

Check the test format ahead of time: the number of questions, the type (multiple choice, free response, etc.), and the time limit. Then create a plan for working through them. For example, if you have 30 minutes to take a 60-question test, your limit is 30 seconds per question. Spend less time on the questions you know well so that you can take more time on the difficult ones.

If you have time to take several practice tests, take the first one open book, with no time limit. Work through the questions at your own pace and make sure you fully understand them. Gradually work up to taking a test under test conditions: sit at a desk with all study materials put away and set a timer. Pace yourself to make sure you finish the test with time to spare and go back to check your answers if you have time.

After each test, check your answers. On the questions you missed, be sure you understand why you missed them. Did you misread the question (tests can use tricky wording)? Did you forget the information? Or was it something you hadn't learned? Go back and study any shaky areas that the practice tests reveal.

Taking these tests not only helps with your grade, but also aids in combating test anxiety. If you're already used to the test conditions, you're less likely to worry about it, and working through tests until you're scoring well gives you a confidence boost. Go through the practice tests until you feel comfortable, and then you can go into the test knowing that you're ready for it.

Test Tips

On test day, you should be confident, knowing that you've prepared well and are ready to answer the questions. But aside from preparation, there are several test day strategies you can employ to maximize your performance.

First, as stated before, get a good night's sleep the night before the test (and for several nights before that, if possible). Go into the test with a fresh, alert mind rather than staying up late to study.

Try not to change too much about your normal routine on the day of the test. It's important to eat a nutritious breakfast, but if you normally don't eat breakfast at all, consider eating just a protein bar. If you're a coffee drinker, go ahead and have your normal coffee. Just make sure you time it so that the caffeine doesn't wear off right in the middle of your test. Avoid sugary beverages, and drink enough water to stay hydrated but not so much that you need a restroom break 10 minutes into the test. If your test isn't first thing in the morning, consider going for a walk or doing a light workout before the test to get your blood flowing.

Allow yourself enough time to get ready, and leave for the test with plenty of time to spare so you won't have the anxiety of scrambling to arrive in time. Another reason to be early is to select a good seat. It's helpful to sit away from doors and windows, which can be distracting. Find a good seat, get out your supplies, and settle your mind before the test begins.

When the test begins, start by going over the instructions carefully, even if you already know what to expect. Make sure you avoid any careless mistakes by following the directions.

Then begin working through the questions, pacing yourself as you've practiced. If you're not sure on an answer, don't spend too much time on it, and don't let it shake your confidence. Either skip it and come back later, or eliminate as many wrong answers as possible and guess among the remaining ones. Don't dwell on these questions as you continue—put them out of your mind and focus on what lies ahead.

Be sure to read all of the answer choices, even if you're sure the first one is the right answer. Sometimes you'll find a better one if you keep reading. But don't second-guess yourself if you do immediately know the answer. Your gut instinct is usually right. Don't let test anxiety rob you of the information you know.

If you have time at the end of the test (and if the test format allows), go back and review your answers. Be cautious about changing any, since your first instinct tends to be correct, but make sure you didn't misread any of the questions or accidentally mark the wrong answer choice. Look over any you skipped and make an educated guess.

At the end, leave the test feeling confident. You've done your best, so don't waste time worrying about your performance or wishing you could change anything. Instead, celebrate the successful completion of this test. And finally, use this test to learn how to deal with anxiety even better next time.

Review Video: Test Anxiety
Visit mometrix.com/academy and enter code: 100340

Important Qualification

Not all anxiety is created equal. If your test anxiety is causing major issues in your life beyond the classroom or testing center, or if you are experiencing troubling physical symptoms related to your anxiety, it may be a sign of a serious physiological or psychological condition. If this sounds like your situation, we strongly encourage you to seek professional help.

Online Resources

Due to our efforts to try to keep this book to a manageable length, we've created a link that will give you access to all of your online resources:

mometrix.com/resources719/crtrrt

It's Your Moment, Let's Celebrate It!

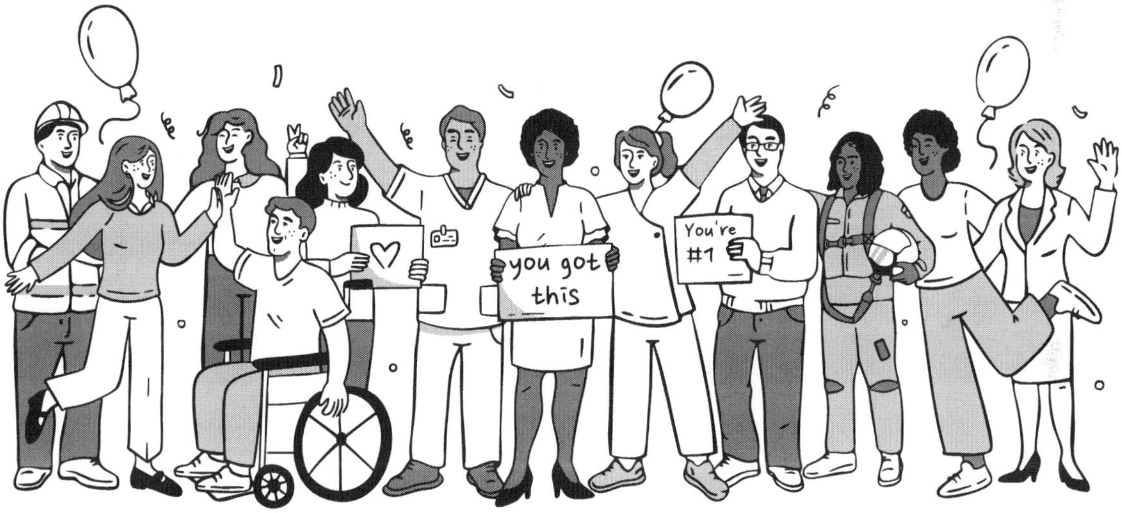

Share your story @mometrixtestpreparation